D0066394

GUIDE TO
Rotational
Atherectomy

MARK REISMAN, M.D.

DIRECTOR, CARDIOVASCULAR RESEARCH

DIRECTOR, CARDIAC CATHETERIZATION LABORATORY

SWEDISH MEDICAL CENTER

SEATTLE, WASHINGTON

PHYSICIANS' PRESS

BIRMINGHAM, MICHIGAN

GUIDE TO
Rotational Atherectomy

Author: Mark Reisman, M.D.
Director of Cardiovascular Research
Swedish Medical Center
Seattle, Washington

Editor: Verna Harms, RN, Ph.D.
Swedish Medical Center
Seattle, Washington

Designer & Illustrator: Brian D. Self
Freelance Designer
Bothell, Washington
e-mail: brianself@earthlink.net

Product Photographer: Don Mason
Don Mason Photography
80 South Jackson
Seattle, Washington

Publisher: Physicians' Press
555 South Woodward Ave., Suite 1409
Birmingham, Michigan 48009
Tel: (248) 645-6443
Fax: (248) 642-4949
web: http://www.physicianspress.com

Printer: K/P Corporation
Seattle, Washington

All right reserved. No part of this publication may be reproduced or transmitted in any form or by any means, electronic or mechanical, including photocopying, recording, or any information storage and retrieval system, without prior written permission from the publisher.

All trademarks mentioned in this book are property of their respective companies.

Copyright © 1997, Physicians' Press

Printed in the United States of America
ISBN 1-890114-02-2

Preface

The evolution of an idea to a tangible medical device requires a combination of a genius and inexhaustible energy, characteristics that just began to describe David C. Auth, Ph.D., the inventor of the Rotablator system. Dr. Auth identified the limitations of the existing methods of percutaneous revascularization and created a device that has and will continue to benefit patients with vascular disease. The path from the "garage" to use in the cardiac catheterization laboratory has been arduous. The effort has taken an orchestrated commitment from many individuals, some of whom I had the pleasure to work with including talented engineers, Tom Clement and Mike Intelkofer, as well as Louise Myers who managed regulatory issues. They have been with David Auth since the beginning, working with some of the rudimentary prototypes and have made significant contributions to the development of the Rotablator system.

The vision had to be realized by others. Businessmen such as Lewis C. Pell, having met with Dr. Auth had the foresight to recognize the utility of this unique device and helped create the entity formerly known as Heart Technology, Inc. The company brought together a mosaic of individuals, all with energy and drive to see that a safe and effective product was delivered to physicians treating vascular disease. I worked closely with many of these individuals including Alan Levy, Karl Mosch, Bill Scott, Walter Blair, David Stiehr and Lisa Zindel. They and many others spent an enormous amount of time and energy to "launch" the Rotablator system into the medical community. Their efforts resulted in creating a certification course that has become the model for the industry. These courses were conducted initially at Washington Hospital Center with Dr. Martin B. Leon and his associates as well as in San Diego where I had the pleasure of working with two superb interventional cardiologists, Dr. Maurice Buchbinder and Dr. Richard Fortuna. I had the opportunity to do my interventional training with Dr. Maurice Buchbinder who, with intelligence and extraordinary skills in the catheterization laboratory, created the platform for the application of the device that we continue to refine and optimize. Several other interventionalists have made considerable contributions to rotational atherectomy and to the review of this manuscript. They include Dr. Gregory Braden, Dr. Samin Sharma, Dr. Ted Feldman and Dr. Patrick Whitlow. I would also like to thank Dr. Mark Freed and Dr. Robert Safian of Physicians' Press for their assistance in the publication of this book.

Finally, if asked again to "write a book" focused on an emerging technology my answer would probably be, no. In contrast to climbing a mountain when ultimately you reach the summit, with a new technology the summit is never established, basic tenets change, experience is gained and thus the book continues to undergo yet another revision. During this "climb" I had two distinguished partners. Verna Harms, whose intelligence, attention to detail and incredible patience allowed me to continually revise the manuscript so that the state of the art is available to the reader.

The other is Brian Self. Brian is one of those magical people who can take a concept and a blank computer screen, and create an image or graphic that makes the complex simple to understand. I am truly grateful for the energy they put into this book. I hope that this book will guide the reader into safe and effective treatment using the Rotablator system.

Dedication

Dedicated to my loving family, my brother Lonny whose gentle hand so often has helped guide me, my sister Hillary, for her passion and energy and my mother Elaine, for the love and commitment to her children which allowed us to strive and realize our dreams.

In memory of our beloved father William Reisman.

Notice

The explosive growth of new equipment and drug therapy has resulted in the rapid evolution and acceptance of practice patterns often based on retrospective non-randomized data and personal experience. Their ultimate role will require close inspection of prospective randomized trials. The clinical recommendations set forth in this book are those of the author; they are offered as *general guidelines only and are not to be construed as absolute indications.* In addition, not all drug or device usages described in this manual have been accepted by the U.S. Food and Drug Administration (USFDA). The use of any drug should be preceded by a careful review of the package insert, which provides indications and dosages as approved by the USFDA. The reader is advised to consult the package insert before using any therapeutic agent. The authors and publisher disclaim responsibility for adverse effects resulting from omissions or undetected errors.

Contents

Appendix

References

Overview of the Rotablator System

Chapter 1

Overview of Rotablator System Components

The Rotablator® system (Figure 1.1) was invented by David C. Auth, Ph.D., P.E. (Boston Scientific Corporation, Northwest Technology Center, Inc., Redmond, Washington) and developed over 13 years. The Rotablator system includes a nickel plated brass elliptical burr coated on the leading edge with diamonds 20–30 μ in diameter (Figure 1.2). Approximately 5 μ of the diamond chips protrude from the nickel plating to form the abrasive surface that ablates atherosclerotic plaque. The burr is attached to a long, flexible driveshaft with a central core with clearance for a 0.009" stainless steel guidewire. The driveshaft is housed in a 4.3 Fr Teflon® sheath and connected to a turbine driven by compressed air or nitrogen. The sheath protects the arterial tissue from potential injury caused by the spinning driveshaft and provides a conduit, delivering fluid (flush) at a rate of 7 cc/min. when the system is nonactivated and 13 cc/min. when the system is activated.

The rotational speed is regulated by air pressure, which is activated with a foot pedal. Depressing the foot pedal initiates rotation of the burr and activates a locking system to prevent the coaxial guidewire from spinning while the burr is rotating. The rpm are measured via a fiber optic light probe (tachometer) and displayed on the console. The console also indicates the time lapsed during a treatment. The speed is generally maintained between

Figure 1.1

Rotablator® System

The components of the Rotablator system include the console, the advancer and the wireClip.

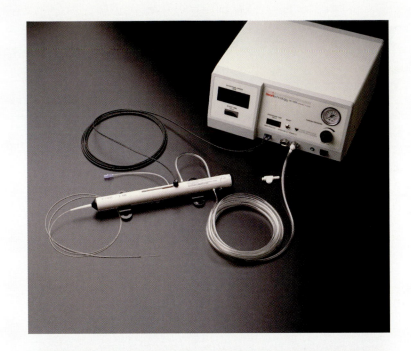

Figure 1.2

Rotablator Burr

A magnified view of the Rotablator burr shows the diamond chips on the distal end and a smooth proximal surface. Rotational energy is delivered to the burr by the driveshaft. The clear sheath shields surrounding vessel tissue from the rotating driveshaft and the accompanying heat. The sheath also serves as a conduit for fluid delivery. The guidewire threads through the burr and the driveshaft and appears distal to the burr in the photo.

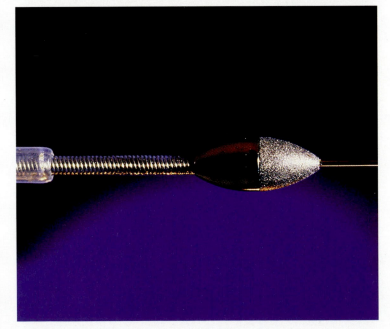

140,000 to 180,000 rpm during treatments, depending on the burr size.

The burr is positioned proximal to the lesion and the advancer knob is used to move the burr forward to engage the lesion. Burrs are available for coronary use in 1.25, 1.50, 1.75, 2.0, 2.15, 2.25, 2.38 and 2.50 mm sizes. Larger sizes are available for peripheral vascular applications.

Four types of guidewires are currently available. The original guidewire, Type C, is a 0.009" stainless steel wire 325 cm long with a 3.7 cm flexible 0.017" diameter platinum radiopaque tip. The clearance between the inner lumen of the burr and the guidewire is 0.001". The Type A wire is similar to the Type C except that the inner core extends to the distal end of the guidewire and it has a 2.7 cm platinum radiopaque tip. Extension of the stainless steel to the distal tip adds further stiffness and the shorter segment of platinum is beneficial in vessels with limited distal beds. In response to suggestions from interventional cardiologists, guidewires with improved tracking and steering characteristics have been developed. The RotaWire™ guidewires are 325 cm long transitional guidewires which taper from 0.009" to 0.005" in the distal end and have, 0.014" diameter, short radiopaque, platinum tips. Operators are presently gaining experience with the RotaWire guidewires to determine the optimal strategy for selection.

The distal platinum tip of the guidewire must be positioned beyond the lesion site since the burr cannot be advanced over this larger segment. A wireClip™ torquer is attached to the proximal end of the guidewire, preventing it from spinning when the brake defeat is activated during withdrawal of the burr (during the exchange procedure). The wireClip is also used as a torquing device.

Based on present guiding catheter technology, the 1.25, 1.50, 1.75, 2.0 and 2.15 mm burrs can be accommodated with an 8 Fr; 2.25 and 2.38 mm burrs with large lumen 9 Fr; and 2.50 mm burrs with a 10 Fr guiding catheter. The inner diameter of guide catheters

Rotablator Guidewires

Type C
- 0.009" diameter
- 3.7 cm long platinum tip
- Soft tip
- 0.017" diameter tip
- 325 cm length

Type A
- 0.009" diameter
- 2.7 cm long platinum tip
- Stiff tip
- 325 cm length

RotaWire™ Floppy
- Tapers in diameter from 0.009" to 0.007" to 0.005" in the distal 44 cm
- 2.2 cm long platinum tip
- Soft tip
- 0.014" diameter tip
- 325 cm length

RotaWire™ Extra Support
- Tapers in diameter from 0.009" to 0.005" in distal 5 cm
- 2.8 cm long platinum tip
- Soft tip
- 0.014" diameter tip
- 325 cm length

(See Appendix Figures 4 and 5 for design details page 270–1.)

Figure 1.3

Differential Cutting

The principle of differential cutting allows the Rotablator to ablate diseased tissue (inelastic), and deflect from healthy tissue (elastic).

A) Elastic Tissue
Normal vascular tissue has elastic properties that allow it to deflect away from the advancing diamonds of the rotating burr.

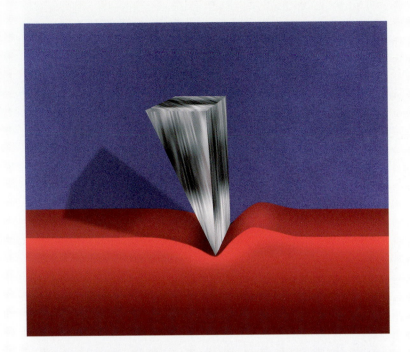

B) Inelastic Tissue
The diamond crystal chips on the distal end of the Rotablator burr cut inelastic tissue during rotation. Unlike healthy tissue, fatty (soft) and calcified (hard) diseased tissue have inelastic properties which prevents deflection away from the advancing burr.

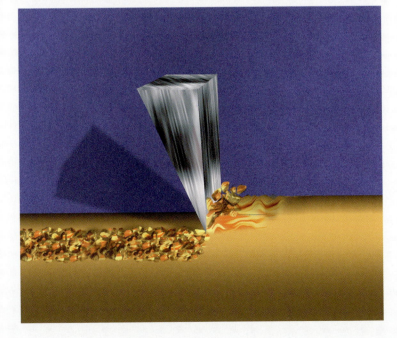

must be 0.004" greater than the burr to provide clearance for device advancement and withdrawal (see Appendix "Coronary Rotablator System Burr Sizes", on page 286).

Physical Principles and Design Characteristics

The Rotablator system is designed as a low-powered rotary sander. This imparts tremendous sensitivity for the operator when advancing the burr in diseased vessels. The slightest load on the system will result in a deceleration of the burr which can be monitored on the digital tachometer display and detected by the sound of the device. A gentle advancement should be employed to "sand" or ablate the plaque.

The two physical principles that govern the operation and effectiveness of the Rotablator system are differential cutting (Figure 1.3) and orthogonal displacement of friction. The Rotablator system's flexibility, tracking and ability to safely and effectively treat arterial obstructions are contingent on these principles.

Differential Cutting

Differential cutting is defined as the ability to selectively ablate one material while sparing and maintaining the integrity of another based on differences in substrate composition.

An example of differential cutting is scraping a knife gently on one's skin and then across a fingernail. The skin is elastic and is able to deflect away from the knife blade unharmed. However, the fingernail is inelastic and will generate fine pulverized debris fragments from the cutting action of the knife blade. Shaving is also an example of differential cutting. A razor will cut inelastic whiskers but spare the healthy underlying elastic skin.

The mechanism of differential cutting is well suited for plaque ablation in the vascular system. Diseased tissue, whether due to calcium, fibrous tissue, fatty deposits or restenotic tissue, is inelastic

Differential Cutting

- Results in preferential cutting of inelastic substrate
- Is functional at low and high speeds

and sanded by the advancing burr. Healthy tissue has elastic properties and therefore can deflect from the cutting edges of the diamond microchips (see Figure 1.3).

Orthogonal Displacement of Friction

The principle of orthogonal displacement of friction, permits the easy passage of the burr through tortuous and diseased segments of the coronary tree. Friction occurs when sliding surfaces are in contact, but it is minimized by a sliding motion perpendicular or orthogonal to the contact surface.

This principle is demonstrated by removal of a cork from a wine bottle. If the cork is twisted as it is pulled, the friction is reduced and the cork can be withdrawn easily. The faster the cork is turned the more easily it is withdrawn. In addition to providing movement through coronary arteries this principle is useful in facilitating the exchange over the guidewire from one burr size to another. At rotational speeds greater than 60,000 rpm, the longitudinal friction vector is virtually eliminated and advancement and withdrawal of the device is unimpeded.

Developmental Studies

Initial investigations of the Rotablator system addressed: 1) the effect of high-speed rotation of an abrasive element on the vascular integrity of normal and abnormal tissue; 2) the impact of microparticulate debris on the myocardium subtended by the vessel; 3) the generation of microcavitations; and 4) the degree of luminal enlargement created by various burr sizes. More recently, the thermal and rheologic effects have been studied.

Effect of High-Speed Rotational Atherectomy on the Vessel Wall

One of the earliest studies to assess the effect of the Rotablator system was performed on 13 New Zealand white rabbits. The rabbits were fed high-cholesterol diets for 2 weeks prior to undergoing iliac artery balloon denudation. At ten weeks contrast angiography revealed greater than 60% arterial narrowing at the

---

Orthogonal Displacement of Friction

- Enables easy navigation through the coronary vasculature
- Effective at speeds greater than 60,000 rpm

denuded segments. These sites were then treated with the Rotablator system at 150,000 rpm.

Following treatment, 11 of the 13 arteries showed a significant angiographic increase in minimal luminal diameter (MLD). The percent diameter stenosis was decreased from 81% ± 9% to 38% ± 22% (mean ± SD, p < 0.001, paired t test). Histological sections demonstrated a smooth, patent lumen, with near total absence of endothelium and various portions of the atheromatous intima missing. The internal elastic lamina were disrupted in some specimens, but medial injury was generally absent. When medial damage was present, it was evidenced by loss of the innermost (luminal) layer of smooth muscle cells. Intimal and medial dissections were not seen.[1]

Ahn et al. performed initial experiments on 68 cadaver arteries with atheromatous lesions involving the superficial femoral, popliteal, and tibial arteries. The specimens were studied angioscopically during treatment and with scanning electron and light microscopy after treatment. The histologic specimens revealed a smooth, highly polished intraluminal surface denuded of intima and endothelial cells (Figure 1.4). Verhoeff-van Gieson stains for elastin revealed that the internal elastic fibers were occasionally disrupted but the outer elastic fibers of the media and adventitial layers were intact. No intimal dissections were observed.[2] Hansen et al. validated the above results with high-speed rotational atherectomy of 11 normal canine coronary arteries. Postmortem examination revealed that treated segments showed extensive intimal loss, with superficial medial damage (which never exceeded 40% of the total medial thickening) and a loss of 20% to 30% of the internal elastic membrane. No perforations were observed.[3]

Finally, Fourrier et al. used the Rotablator system on femoral arteries prior to undergoing femoral-popliteal bypass surgery. The results were consistent with prior studies demonstrating the removal of fibrous and calcified atherosclerotic plaque. The abraded surface was smooth and, importantly, free of thrombus. The endothelium of the adjacent wall was removed and no medial

Figure 1.4 A&B

Microscopy After Treatment

Histologic examination of arteries after treatment with rotational atherectomy reveals a smooth round lumen.

A) Scanning Electron Micrograph

A smooth luminal surface is often created by the diamond-tipped burr of the Rotablator system, as demonstrated by this scanning electronmicrograph.

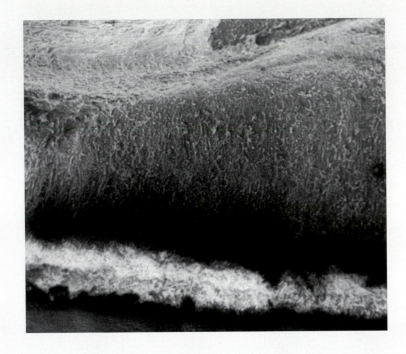

B) Lumen Cross Section

A histological cross section of a vessel treated with the Rotablator reveals a smooth concentric lumen.

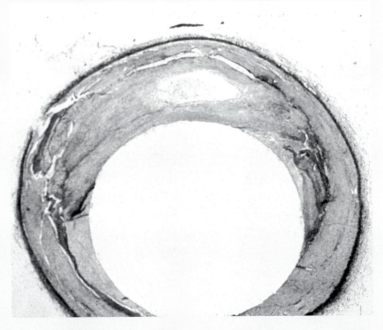

damage was noted. There was absence of dehiscence between plaque and arterial wall. A few surface irregularities were seen in areas where the Rotablator system was used at rotational speeds less than 75,000 rpm.[4]

The advent of intravascular ultrasound and its recent refinement have provided an additional window into the lumen of arterial segments. Mintz et al. analyzed images of 11 patients treated with the Rotablator system and subsequently evaluated with intravascular ultrasound. Four patients demonstrated fissures, one had a dissection, and none had arterial expansion (defined as the area within the external elastic membrane at the angioplasty site greater than that of the proximal reference segment). Using a three-dimensional reconstruction of cross-sectional images, a smooth tubular lumen was observed, especially in areas of densest calcium.[5]

Potkin et al. assessed the outcome of calcified versus noncalcified lesions treated with the Rotablator system and noted no evidence of dissections or arterial expansion in either group. In the calcified group, fewer than half the patients had fissures, while the noncalcified group had no sign of fissures.[6]

Finally, Kovach et al. studied 46 patients with calcified vessels and analyzed lumen and plaque cross-sectional areas using three-dimensional reconstruction of intravascular ultrasound images. Areas treated with high-speed rotational atherectomy had a significant increase in luminal diameter based on a decrease in cross-sectional plaque area. No evidence of vessel expansion was demonstrated, implying that atherectomy, was the mechanism by which larger lumens were obtained.[7]

A concern with high-speed rotational atherectomy is the impact of the burr on sites proximal and distal to the treated segment. Quantitative coronary angiography at 24-hours and at 3- to 6-month follow-up intervals revealed no evidence of changes in luminal dimensions at these sites after treatment suggesting that accelerated atherosclerosis in non-diseased segments does not occur.[8]

Production of Microparticles

The sharp, multifaceted diamond crystals of the Rotablator burr are protuberant pyramids of approximately 5 μ. The sanding process is able to directly cleave chemical bonds by forceful shearing of the molecular structure. This is a mechanical shear in distinction to the shear induced by expanding vesicles of steam produced by laser or electrosurgery. The size of the microparticles liberated from the tissue by the advancing burr is determined by the crystal size and importantly by the pressure applied to the tissue. Light pressure or gentle advancement will result in generation of particles smaller than the diamond size, while heavy pressure to the tissue or aggressive advancement will result in the diamonds deeply penetrating the tissue and producing larger particles. By controlling the amount of forward pressure the physician can influence the depth of cutting and the size of the atheromatous material as it is converted into microparticles (Figure 1.5 and 1.6). This key feature eliminates the need for an aspiration or collection device.

Distribution and Effects of Microparticulate Debris

The effect of the particles produced by the Rotablator procedure has been a major concern since the initial investigations. In one in vitro study, segments of rabbit aorta 3–5 cm in length were treated with rotational atherectomy while undergoing continuous saline perfusion. Examination by Coulter counter revealed that 1.5% to 2.0% of the particles were greater than 10 μ while the average particle size was less than 5 μ.[1] Similar findings were observed when ablating human atherosclerotic iliac arteries where 77% of the particles generated were less than 5 μ and 88% were less than 12 μ, with an average of 10^6 microparticles per milliliter.[9]

Experimental studies to assess in vivo effects used human particulate debris injected into the left circumflex of three dogs. Myocardial blood flow was analyzed using radiolabeled

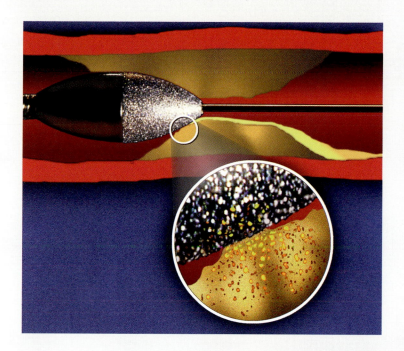

Figure 1.5

Rotary Sander

The Rotablator driveshaft and burr comprise what is basically a low-powered rotary sander. The low-torque design imparts tremendous sensitivity to the operator as the device is advanced through diseased vessel segments. The slightest load on the burr will result in a drop in rpm.

Gentle advancement should be employed to "sand" or ablate the plaque into microparticles.

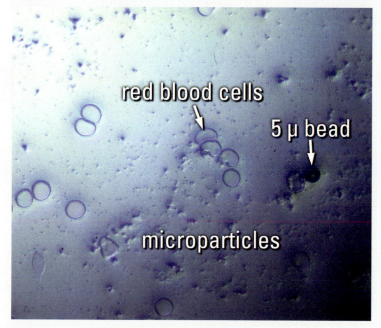

red blood cells

5 μ bead

microparticles

Figure 1.6

Microparticle Debris

The Rotablator generates microparticle debris. A 5 μ bead establishes size of the microparticles in the image.

microspheres. In two dogs there was no detectable change in myocardial blood flow after a 32 cc injection of noncalcified particulate debris. The third dog was subjected to large boluses of 42 cc and 96 cc of heavily calcified debris which reduced myocardial blood flow by 50% and 100% of control values, respectively. These quantities are estimated to be 10 to 30 times the volume produced from human coronary lesions.[9]

Particulate debris was further investigated by subjecting human cadaveric lower extremity vessels to high-speed rotational atherectomy and labeling the effluent with technetium-99. These radiolabeled particles were then injected into the common femoral artery of five dogs and scanned by nuclear scintigraphy. The study demonstrated that a minority of particles lodged in the lower extremities while the majority passed through the circulation and were cleared by the liver, lung, and spleen.[2] In a similar experiment, debris from rotational atherectomy on human cadaveric coronary arteries was collected and injected into the left anterior descending (LAD) artery of dogs. There were no significant changes in heart rate, left ventricular end diastolic pressure, systolic blood pressure, coronary blood flow or coronary flow reserve. Regional myocardial function was minimally reduced for 30 minutes after injection of the debris. After 60 minutes, complete recovery was observed. Pathologic sections of the canine hearts revealed evidence of limited areas of necrotic myofibers of single cells and clusters of 3 to 4 cells.[10]

The effects of microparticles produced by rotational atherectomy in human clinical studies were investigated with positron emission tomography (PET). Myocardial perfusion was evaluated in nine patients using N-13 ammonia. In all patients there was no evidence of procedure-related infarction by ECG, CPK elevation, or clinical history. In two patients where myocardial perfusion was normal by PET on polar maps, there was no significant change post-therapy. In seven patients with impaired baseline myocardial perfusion, the perfusion improved after treatment. Concomitant left ventricular function was analyzed using echocardiography. Four patients had normal function which was unchanged post-procedure, and, of five patients with hypokinesis, four demonstrated no change and one had improvement.[11]

Finally, Pavlides et al. studied 17 patients undergoing rotational atherectomy with ECG, hemodynamic monitoring, and simultaneous transesophageal echocardiography. The results showed that the hemodynamic parameters and global left ventricular function remained unchanged during rotational atherectomy. Regional wall motion function in the distribution of the target coronary artery (assessed by wall motion score) was also shown to be unaffected during treatment.[12] In contrast, Huggins et al. demonstrated a transient (30–40 minutes) decrease in wall motion; the dominant mechanism was presumed to be myocardial stunning.[13,14]

In summary, these investigational studies suggest that possible damage produced by the distal embolization of microparticles has not been realized in the majority of experimental trials. Extrapolation of these findings to the clinical setting would suggest that ablation of plaque with the Rotablator system results in reliably small to moderate amounts of distal debris embolization and should be accompanied by minimal effects on the myocardium subtended by the vessel.

Microcavitations Produced with the Rotablator System

One unresolved question is whether microcavitations are formed during high-speed rotational atherectomy. The critical speed for dissolving gas-forming bubbles (microcavitations) in blood is 14.7 m/sec. A 2.0 mm burr operating at 160,000 rpm would rotate at a speed of 16.7 m/sec., and would establish the conditions necessary for production of microcavitations.

Zotz et al. studied the in vivo and in vitro production of microcavitations. Transthoracic and transesophageal echocardiograms were obtained before and after treatment from nine patients treated with the Rotablator system. Treatment intervals lasted 10 seconds and were interrupted by one to two minutes of recovery. None of the patients experienced a decrease in regional ejection fraction during or after rotational atherectomy. With the onset of high-speed rotational atherectomy, transient enhancement of echo contrast occurred in the area of myocardium supplied by the treated artery and disappeared immediately after burr rotation was stopped. The debris was unlikely the source of the myocardial contrast enhancement, because the opacification was transient and occurred prior to advancing the device. In vitro experimentation to study bubble size using high-speed rotational atherectomy in fresh whole blood measured a mean bubble size of 90 μ ± 33 μ. The bubble dimensions are large when compared to the 7 μ mean size of red blood cells. The collapse time of these cavitation bubbles was calculated to be very short, in the range of 10 seconds.[15]

In summary, high-speed rotational atherectomy may result in the formation of microcavitations that are relatively large but collapse quickly. To date there is no direct evidence that indicates deleterious effects. However, further studies evaluating the role of microcavitations in the clinical setting may have technical implications on rotational speed and duration of treatment.

Efficiency of Rotational Atherectomy
The efficiency of debulking with the Rotablator system has been investigated using quantitative coronary angiography. Early studies using quantitative coronary angiography on 109 patients demonstrated that a predictable minimum luminal diameter (MLD) can be achieved across the spectrum of burr sizes (ranging from 1.75 to 2.25 mm). Expressing this MLD as a burr ratio (MLD/burr size), the Rotablator achieved immediate results of 0.72 ± 0.19 of the burr selected (i.e., a 2.0 mm burr predicted a MLD of approximately 1.4 mm). When these lesion sites were then

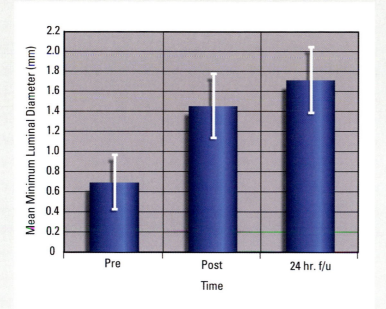

Figure 1.7

Luminal Diameter Gains

Minimal luminal diameter in patients undergoing rotational atherectomy measured before, immediately post-procedure and at 24-hours post-procedure.

MLD shown as mean ± standard deviations (n=186).

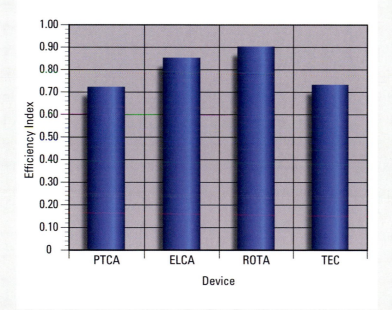

Figure 1.8

Device Efficiency

The Rotablator burr is able to create a lumen that is 90% of the diameter of the burr (i.e. 90% efficient) compared to 72–85% device efficiency for PTCA, ELCA and TEC.

measured at 24-hour follow-up, the burr ratio increased to 0.84 ± 0.15. The increased luminal diameter at 24 hours was confirmed by analyzing a cohort of 186 patients who were studied with quantitative coronary angiography before, immediately after, and during follow-up the next day (Figure 1.7). On average the luminal dimensions had increased at 24 hours. Analysis by patient of the MLD, comparing post-procedure to 24 hours, revealed that 17% had lost > 0.05 mm, 10% were within ± 0.05 mm and 73% had gained > 0.05 mm. This late gain may be due to resolution of vasospasm or to an increased blood flow.[16]

More recent studies (Figure 1.8) demonstrate that the gain achieved immediately post-rotational atherectomy can approximate a cutting efficiency of 0.9. This compares favorably with other methods of percutaneous revascularization.[17]

Mintz et al., using intravascular ultrasound found that when the minimum lumen diameter was divided by the largest burr used, the ratio ranged from 0.93 to 1.45 (1.19 ± 0.19) for stand-alone procedures and 1.02 to 1.56 (1.30 ± 0.15) (p = ns) for Rotablator plus adjunct balloon angioplasty.[7] In this study, there appears to be a trend towards a lumen in excess of the burr size. This trend was present regardless of the amount of plaque or use of adjunct balloon angioplasty. One possible explanation is that once the plaque is ablated, the vessel becomes "unbound" and the vasomotor function is restored. Another possibility could be due to an eccentric guidewire orientation which can result in preferential ablation of the plaque, causing greater cross-sectional ablation area than the burr size (see Chapter 3 "Guidewire Selection and Placement", page 48).

Thermal Effects of Rotational Atherectomy
Thermal injury due to heat has been identified by studying tissue specimens of patients treated with rotational atherectomy followed by directional atherectomy.[18] In order to assess the thermal changes of rotational atherectomy, model in vitro and in vivo systems have been studied.[19]

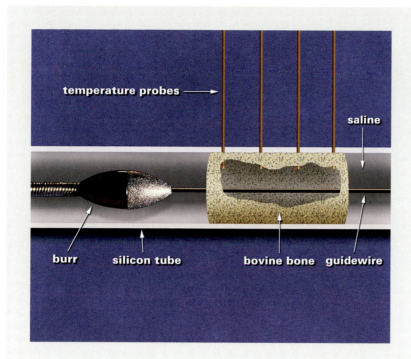

temperature probes ──→

saline

burr **silicon tube** **bovine bone** **guidewire**

Figure 1.9

Thermal Tests

This experimental apparatus measures heat generated by the burr. The tests utilize bovine bone fitted with temperature probes to take measurements during ablation using various techniques.

Using an experimental design that included 12 mm cylinders derived from bovine femurs with 0.35 mm cored lumens to permit passage of the Rotablator guidewire, 4 thermal probes were placed at intervals of 3 mm to assess temperature changes as the burr engaged that segment of bone (Figure 1.9). With continuous saline infusion at body temperature, 2.0 mm burrs were advanced through the model and simultaneous data acquisition included revolutions per minute (rpm) and temperature. Two methods of advancement of the burr were applied, either a continuous advancement through the entire segment or an intermittent or oscillating technique which consisted of a 2 second engagement of the bone followed by a 2 second withdrawal in order to permit reestablishment of antegrade flow. Both methods were tested using an aggressive ablation technique with excessive decelerations (14,000–18,000 rpm) or a gentle advancement technique which limited decelerations to 4,000–6,000 rpm. The results are shown in

Heat Generation

Heat generation depends on the ablation technique. An intermittent or oscillating technique generates the least amount of heat when applied with minimal decelerations.

- CAED: Continuous Ablation Excessive Decelerations of 14,000–18,000 rpm
- CAMD: Continuous Ablation Minimal Decelerations of 4,000–6,000 rpm
- IAED: Intermittent Ablation Excessive Decelerations of 14,000–18,000 rpm
- IAMD: Intermittent Ablation Minimal Decelerations of 4,000–6,000 rpm

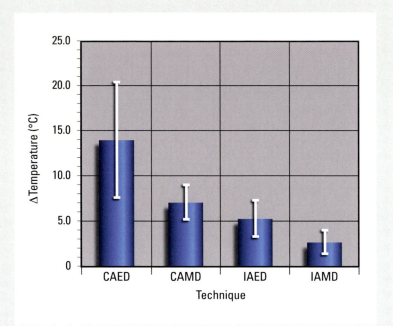

Figure 1.10. Subsequent experimentation to assess the impact of heat generation using gentle vs. aggressive advancement was accomplished with an in vivo miniswine model. The femoral artery was exposed and cradled in a constricting sheath containing thermal probes (Figure 1.11). The probes were in contact with the adventicia of the artery and simultaneous recording of the rpm and temperature were acquired as the burr was advanced through the cradled segment. The burr was activated proximal to the constricting sheath and was either advanced aggressively with significant decelerations of 10,000–15,000 rpm or gently with decelerations ranging between 5,000–9,000 rpm with corresponding temperature elevations of 11.3 ± 6.2°C and 4.1 ± 1.2°C, respectively (p < 0.05).[20]

The literature is replete with studies demonstrating the association of thermal injury with smooth muscle proliferation,

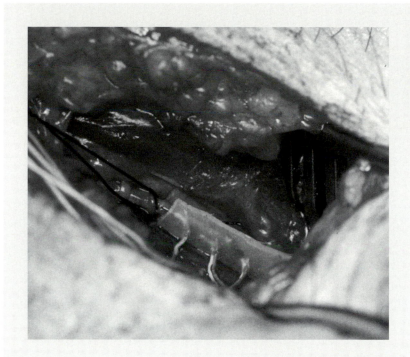

Figure 1.11

In Vivo Thermal Apparatus

To measure the thermal effects of rotational atherectomy in vivo, the femoral artery of a miniswine was cradled in a sheath with constricting thermal probes. As the Rotablator burr was advanced through the sheath the temperature was recorded.

high restenosis rates, RBC aggregation, and platelet activation.[22-26] Interestingly, the "benchmark" studies of rotational atherectomy[27-29] applied the old recommendations which included activating all burr sizes at 180,000–200,000 rpm with a 10% deceleration as the burr crosses the lesion (19,000–20,000 rpm) as acceptable.

As the secondary effects of rotational atherectomy, especially thermal injury, have been understood, techniques such as minimizing decelerations have been advocated. Whether the technique modifications will impact immediate clinical outcome and long-term restenosis have yet to be determined.

Hematologic Impact of Rotational Atherectomy

The high-speed rotating burr establishes a shear field in the blood affecting both erythrocytes and platelets (Figure 1.12). An

Figure 1.12

Blood Aggregates

Porcine blood was exposed to a rotating burr, resulting in platelet aggregation and red blood cell crenation.

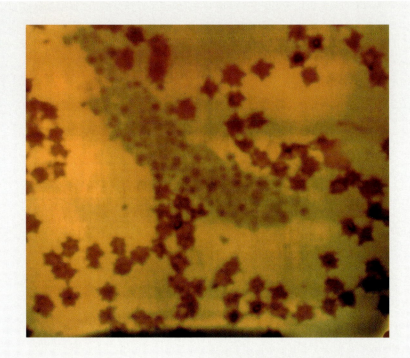

Table 1.1

Platelet Aggregation

Rotational speeds influence platelet aggregation, with slower speed resulting in a significantly smaller number of platelet aggregates.

Rotational Speed	Platelet Aggregates > 20 μm/ml blood
180,000 rpm	7,137 ± 1,993
140,000 rpm	2,255 ± 605
Control	633 ± 258

*n=8 for group, p < 0.0001 for all groups

investigation using porcine blood exposed to the spinning burr in an in vitro model demonstrated platelet aggregation as measured by optical microscopy.[21] The number of aggregates was affected by the speed of the burr and differed significantly at the predesignated speeds of 180,000 and 140,000 (Table 1.1). Larger platelet aggregates, $\geq 60\ \mu$ in diameter, were seen in 8/8 samples run at 180,000 rpm and in only one sample (1/8) with a speed of 140,000 rpm. Plasma free hemoglobin was 429 ± 168 mg/dl vs. 88 ± 44 mg/dl, and the activated clotting time was 237 ± 19 sec. vs. 493 ± 179 sec. for the 180,000 vs. the 140,000 rpm groups respectively. Based on these results, a clinical registry has been designed to assess whether lower speeds will have a beneficial effect on patient outcomes.

Summary

These studies establish the foundation for understanding the mechanism of rotational atherectomy. In a majority of cases, the microparticulate debris passes benignly through the coronary circulation and is cleared by the reticular endothelial system. The resultant lumen is often smooth and free of dissections. More recent studies have shown that heat generation and thermal injury can be minimized by gentle advancement of the device avoiding significant decelerations. Platelet aggregation is dependent on burr speed and may be open to modulation by assessing the effectiveness of the device at lower speeds. The following chapter reviews clinical studies of rotational atherectomy and provides preliminary evidence that technique modifications to minimize heat generation and platelet activation may impact outcomes.

Overview of Clinical Data

Chapter 2

Rotational atherectomy prior to release in the United States was evaluated in a multicenter registry which resulted in FDA approval in May, 1993. The following section includes the results of the multicenter registry as well as substudies and single-center experiences. The results represent a time point in a continuum in the evolution of a device that has undergone dynamic change. The change has not been in the design of the Rotablator system, but rather the technique with which it is applied.

Results of the Multicenter Registry

The multicenter investigation of the Rotablator system began in 1988, with 18 centers. The initial enrollment included patients whose anatomy was deemed suboptimal for standard balloon angioplasty, and patients previously treated with balloon angioplasty who presented with restenosis or had failure to achieve an adequate result. Later, as data accrued with favorable results, and the investigators' experience and comfort with device increased, more complex lesions were approached including heavily calcified lesions, lesions greater than 10 mm in length, eccentric lesions and total or subtotal chronic occlusions.

Patients with acute myocardial infarction were excluded as were patients with post-infarction angina since, mechanistically, thrombus is an inadequate substrate for the device. Also excluded were saphenous vein bypass grafts, lesions > 25 mm in length, and patients with ejection fractions < 30%. Each patient gave informed consent using the protocol approved by their respective institutional review board.

The multicenter registry included a total of 2,953 procedures involving 3,717 lesions and remains the benchmark study of rotational atherectomy until the ongoing clinical trials are completed. The mean age of the patients was 63 ± 11 years (SD) with the majority being males (71.4%). The clinical antecedents (Figure 2.1) consisted of a majority of patients with stable angina and multivessel disease. Slightly less than half had previous myocardial infarction or unstable angina. The lesions were distributed with a predominance in the LAD (LAD 47%, RCA 30%, circumflex 19%, protected left main 3%). When assessing by lesion morphology the majority of lesions were classified as AHA/ACC Type B (17% A, 66% B, 17% C), with 49% calcified, 69% eccentric, 28% at bifurcations, and 66% de novo lesions (Figure 2.2). The

Figure 2.1

Patient Characteristics in the Multicenter Registry

Abbreviations:
- MVD= multivessel disease
- Chol = hypercholesterolemia
- HTN = hypertension
- USA = unstable angina
- MI = prior myocardial infarction
- DM = diabetes mellitus
- CABG = prior bypass surgery

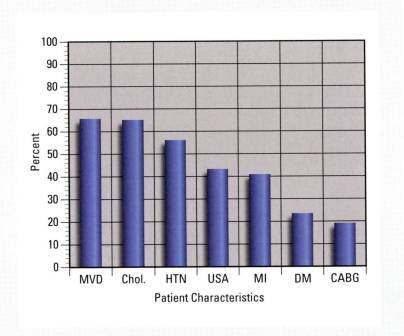

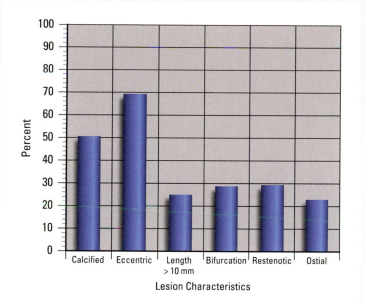

Figure 2.2

Lesion Morphology

In the multicenter registry, 50% of lesions had moderate to severe calcification and 25% of lesions were greater than 10 mm in length.

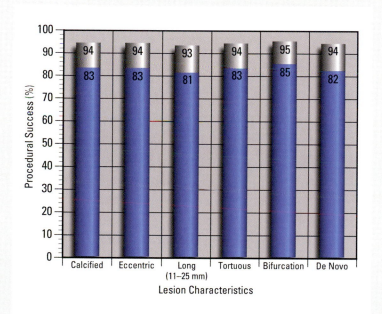

Figure 2.3

Procedural Success

Independent of lesion characteristics the procedural success, defined as < 50% residual stenosis in the absence of death, Q-wave myocardial infarction or emergency bypass surgery, was 81% to 85% with rotational atherectomy alone (blue bar) and increased to over 93% (gray bar) after adjunctive PTCA.

Figure 2.4

Angiographic Diameter by QCA

Minimum luminal diameter at baseline (pre), 24-hours post-procedure, and 6-months post-procedure of patients treated with rotational atherectomy alone or with adjunctive balloon angioplasty.

Blue columns represent mean lumen diameters, gray bars represent standard deviations (n = 92).

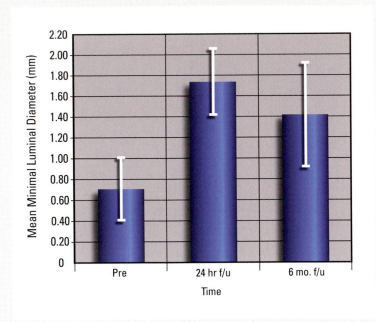

lesions were less than 10 mm long in 76% of the cases, and between 11 to 25 mm long in 24% of the cases.

The procedural success rate was 85% with the Rotablator system alone, and increased to 95% with adjunctive balloon angioplasty. A wide variety of lesions were treated with similar procedural success (Figure 2.3). Major clinical complications included: 1.2% Q-wave myocardial infarction (MI), 2.5% coronary bypass surgery, and 1.0% death.[67] Other complications included CK elevation (non-Q-wave MI) in 6.1% of the patients. Angiographic complications included: 0.7% perforation, 13.7% dissection, and 1.1% abrupt closure post-procedure. Restenosis rates were 50% in the 50% of patients who returned for angiographic follow-up. The majority of these patients were symptomatic. Full QCA was performed on 92 patients who under went both 24-hour and 6-month follow-up. Minimum luminal diameter from decreased 1.72 ± 0.32 mm at

24-hours post-procedure to 1.45 ± 0.48 mm at 6 months (Figure 2.4).

Based on the results of the multicenter registry, the Rotablator system received FDA approval for use by interventional cardiologists who had attended and participated in a training course conducted by Boston Scientific Corporation Northwest Technology Center, Inc. (formerly Heart Technology, Inc.). More than 2,000 physicians have completed the certification course and are actively using the device.

Results of Observational Studies

Several studies have presented findings based on examining single-site experiences using rotational atherectomy. One of the central features of these studies is the wide range of success and complications with the device (Tables 2.1, 2.2 and 2.3). This variation is most probably a result of the heterogeneity in technique of the initial investigators. The improved results seen in later studies and in more complex lesion subsets is a testimony to the evolution of the technique and greater comfort with the device.

Restenosis rates are difficult to interpret. These rates rely on angiographic follow-up of less than 60% of the patients in the multicenter trial and on differing definitions of restenosis in the various studies. In addition, Rotablator technique (maximal safe debulking) and post-Rotablator balloon strategies (high- vs. low-pressure inflations) may impact restenosis rates and need further study.

The largest trial comparing rotational atherectomy to other devices in a randomized design is the Excimer Laser vs. Rotablator vs. Balloon Trial (ERBAC).[36] The lesions treated were AHA/ACC classes B2 or C. Rotational atherectomy, compared to balloon or laser, had a significantly lower rate of major complications with a smaller residual stenosis and fewer lesions requiring crossover to other techniques (Table 2.4). In the 6-month follow-up, the incidence of death and Q-wave myocardial infarction were not different. The

Table 2.1

Clinical Outcome After Rotational Atherectomy

Abbreviations:
- Major complications: Death, emergent bypass surgery or Q-wave MI.
- Non-QMI: CK > 2x normal with positive CK-MB.
- Rest.: Restenosis.
- CTO: Chronic Total Occlusion
- Ca: Moderate to severe calcification
- A, B, C: ACC/AHA lesion classification
- Blanks: Data not available.

Clinical Complications

Study (yr)[ref.]	N	Lesion Type	Major Comp. %	Non-QMI Comp. %	Rest. %
Dietz ('91)[34]	106	B, C with 44 % CTO	1.9	4.7	42
Teirstein ('91)[30]	42	71% > 10 mm	4.0	19	59
Barrione ('93)[31]	166	Complex 63%	2.4	8.4	
Gilmore ('93)[32]	108	N/A	4.6	2.8	
Guerin ('93)[33]	61	B_2 100%	3.2	6.6	
Safian ('93)[29]	104	A 20%, B 76%, C 4%	7.7	2.9	51
Stertzer ('93)[28]	302	A 7.5%, B/C 92.5%	3.6		37
Ellis ('94)[35]	316	A 24%, B 70%, C 6%	3.4	5.7	
Vandormael ('94)[36]	215	B_1 15%, B_2 72%, C 13%	2.3		62
Warth ('94)[27]	743	A 27%, B 59%, C 14%	3.4	3.8	38
MacIsaac ('95)[37]	2,161	Ca 50%, Non-Ca 50%	3.5	8.8	

Table 2.2

Angiographically Identified Complications

Abbreviations:
- Perf.: Perforation
- Dis.: Dissection
- Blanks: Data not available

Angiographic Complications

Study[ref.]	N	Abrupt Closure	Slow Flow/ No Reflow	Perf.	Post-Lab Closure	Dis.	Side Branch Occlus.	Severe Spasm
Safian[29]	116	11.2	6.1	0	3.6		1.8	
Dietz[34]	106						1.9	6.6
Barrione[31]	166	1.8						
Guerin[33]	67							4.5
Warth[27]	874	3.1	1.2	0.5	0.9	10.5	0.1	1.6
Ellis[35]	400	5.5	7.6	1.5				
MacIsaac[37]	2,161	3.6		0.7		13.0		

Procedural Success by Lesion Characteristics

Study[ref.]	Number of Lesions	Lesion Type	Procedural Success (%)
MacIsaac[37]	1,078	Ca	94
	1,083	Non-Ca	95
Altmann[38]	675	No/Mild Ca	96
		Mod. Ca	96
		Heavy Ca	92
Vandormael[36]	215	B2 72%; C 13%	91
Reisman[39]	953	< 10 mm	95
	180	11–15 mm	97
	143	15–25 mm	92
Favereau[40]	215	10–20 mm	95
	73	> 20 mm	84
Koller[41]	29	Ostial	93
Popma[42]	105	Ostial	97
Zimarino[43]	69	Ostial	92
Omoigui[44]	145	Chronic Total	91
Reisman[45]	67	Undilatable	97
Brogan[46]	41	Undilatable	90
Rosenblum[47]	41	Undilatable	97
Sievert[48]	32	Undilatable	97
Bass[49]	428	Restenotic	97
Chevalier[50]	123	Angulated	86

Table 2.3

Procedural Success for Differing Lesion Types

High procedural success was obtained for most lesion types. Angulated lesions had the lowest procedural success, most probably due to unfavorable guidewire bias.

incidence of lesion revascularization was higher for rotational atherectomy and laser than for balloon although the differences in angiographic restenosis rates failed to achieve significance.

Recently, the results of Kaplan et al.[51] suggest that the burr-to-artery ratio may influence the target vessel revascularization (Figure 2.5) with either minimal or excessive debulking resulting in a higher incidence of restenosis.

Clinical Trials

Several large multicenter randomized clinical trials are in progress to further explore the effectiveness of rotational atherectomy.

STRATAS (Study to Determine Rotablator and Transluminal Angioplasty Strategy)

STRATAS is a technique trial exploring two potential methods to use the Rotablator system. The design is a multicenter two-arm randomization with a total enrollment of 500 patients. One arm will use an approach of maximal debulking (0.8–0.9 burr-to-artery ratio) with no or low-pressure adjunctive PTCA (less than 1 atm) and compare that to a technique of moderate debulking (≤ 0.75 burr-to-artery ratio) with systematic conventional PTCA. The hypothesis of this trial is that aggressive debulking with minimal stretch or dilation will reduce the progenitors of restenosis. The enrollment phase of STRATAS is completed and shows that in the acute phase both strategies were equally successful with the aggressive strategy using more burrs (2.8 vs. 2.1), having, as expected, a higher burr-to-artery ratio (by QCA 93% vs. 82%) and a longer burr run time (315 vs. 231 sec.).[52] Using chart recorders to determine speed changes during ablation, a substudy of this trial showed that decelerations greater than 5,000 rpm for longer than 10 seconds or decelerations greater than 7,000 rpm for longer than 5 seconds were significant predictors of major cardiac events and CKMB elevation post-procedure (Table 2.5).[53,54] Upon completion of the trial the impact of debulking strategy on restenosis will be available.

	PTCA N=210	ELCA N=195	PTRA N=215	p
B2/C (%)	60/12	68/10	72/13	
Success Before Crossover (%)	80	76	91	< 0.001
Final (%)	36 ± 15	32 ± 15	31 ± 16	< 0.05
Death, QMI, CABG (%)	4.8	6.2	2.3	0.04
Eligible f/u pts.	170	174	191	
f/u rate (%)	77	85	81	NS
Death, QMI (%)	3.1/3.8	0/0.7	2.6/3.2	NS
Lesion revasc. (%)	35	46	46	0.04
Angio. Rest. (%)	54	60	62	NS

Table 2.4

Randomized Trial (ERBAC)

The ERBAC trial was a randomized trial of PTCA vs. Rotablator (Rota) vs. excimer laser (ELCA). Rotablator demonstrated a higher rate of success before crossover and a lower rate of major complications. Angiographic restenosis rate was not different but lesion revascularization occurred more frequently in the Rotablator and laser groups.

Source: Stoerger, et al., Heart Center and Red Cross Hospital, Frankfurt/Main Germany

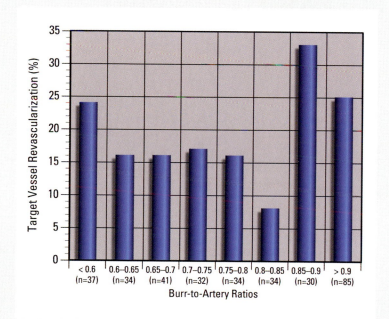

Figure 2.5

Revascularization Based on Burr-to-Artery Ratio

Target vessel revascularization rates may be dependent on the magnitude of debulking, with minimal or excessive debulking resulting in a higher incidence of repeat revascularization procedures. (Number of lesions treated is shown in parenthesis.)

Table 2.5

Technique as a Predictor of Adverse Events

Technique, including decelerations > 5,000 rpm for > 10 sec., predicted major adverse cardiac events (MACE and post-procedure CKMB elevation in a substudy of the STRATAS trial. Final data analysis will determine whether technique predicts restenosis as well.

	MACE p	CKMB p
Deceleration > 5,000 rpm > 10 seconds	< 0.03	< 0.005
Deceleration > 7,000 rpm > 5 seconds	< 0.02	< 0.008
Any deceleration > 10,000 rpm	< 0.96	< 0.96
Mean time per run (s)	< 0.71	< 0.0001
Total rotational atherectomy time (s)	< 0.61	< 0.0001
Total RA time > 300 seconds	0.02	< 0.002

Table 2.6

Effect of ReoPro on CK Elevation

A retrospective single-site experience demonstrated that the use of ReoPro, a glycoprotein IIb/IIIa inhibitor, decreased the incidence of CK elevation after Rotablator procedures. Major clinical complications were not affected. (CABG 0% vs. 1%; Q-MI 0% vs. 0%; death 0% vs. 0%; bleeding 2% vs. 0%; Reopro vs. control p=NS.

- ReoPro = Rotational atherectomy procedures performed with ReoPro (bolus and infusion)
- Control = Rotational atherectomy procedures performed without ReoPro

	ReoPro N=100	Control N=100	P value N=100
Peak CK	145 ± 13	238 ± 20	0.02
1–3xNL	10%	17%	0.15
> 3xNL	3%	9%	0.07
Any Abn. CK	13%	26%	0.02

DART (Dilation vs. Ablation Revascularization Trial)

DART is a two-arm multicenter randomized design with a primary endpoint of clinical and angiographic restenosis. The DART trial will compare rotational atherectomy with or without adjunctive low-pressure PTCA (less than 1 atm) to conventional PTCA in noncomplex (type A or B1) lesions with reference vessels less than 3.0 mm in diameter. The trial will enroll 500 patients and involve approximately 35 centers.

Rotational Atherectomy with Glycoprotein IIB/IIIA Inhibitors (ReoPro)

The role of rotational atherectomy in inducing platelet aggregation has been described in Chapter 1. The use of ReoPro, a glycoprotein IIb/IIIa inhibitor, to mitigate platelet activation and its effect on procedural success and long-term outcome is unknown. A multicenter registry of rotational atherectomy and ReoPro[55] and a single-center comparison of atherectomy cases with and without ReoPro[56] have demonstrated that ReoPro is safe and that it reduces CK elevation post-procedure (Table 2.6). In the registry of 165 patients treated with rotational atherectomy and ReoPro there were two Q-wave MIs, no bypass surgeries and no deaths. Bleeding complications resulting in transfusion occurred in 3% of patients. The average length of stay was 1.7 days with 88% discharged within 2 days. A CK elevation above normal was experienced by 18% of patients with 6% having CK > 2x normal. A multicenter trial in complex lesions (> 20 mm and/or with moderate to severe calcium) has been organized to study patients treated with ReoPro or placebo during rotational atherectomy to determine in a prospective randomized design whether ReoPro decreases intraprocedural complications such as slow flow or post-procedural CKMB elevations. Secondary endpoints will compare major adverse events and clinical restenosis rates.

Rotational Atherectomy with Adjunctive Stenting (Rotastent)

The synergy of two second-generation devices such as rotational atherectomy and stenting may have a significant role in revascularization, since rotastenting is a true synergy in that rotational atherectomy can increase lesion compliance to allow maximal luminal dimensions post-stenting.

In a retrospective analysis of 178 patients/224 lesions (70% calcified, reference diameter 2.81 ± 0.43 mm) treated with rotational atherectomy followed by stent, procedural success was achieved in 91.9% with an average residual stenosis of $6.1 \pm 19.4\%$ and a target lesion revascularization at > 4 months of 12.5%.[57] Mintz et al. had demonstrated using intravascular ultrasound that rotational atherectomy followed by stent yielded a larger luminal gain (7.3 mm² vs. 5.1 mm²) and smaller residual stenosis than (12% vs. 27%) rotational atherectomy followed by adjunctive balloon angioplasty with no apparent increase in complications.[58] A randomized multicenter trial comparing PTCA-stent to Rotastent in lesions with moderate to severe calcification and/or longer than 20 mm is being designed. The trial will investigate whether rotational atherectomy prior to stenting portends an advantage in stent delivery, deployment and long-term outcome. Intravascular ultrasound will be an interactive component in the trial to assess stent deployment at various predetermined pressures.

TWISTER (Trial of Within Stent Treatment of Endoluminal Restenosis)

The management of stent restenosis (intrastent restenosis) will become an important issue in the future with the proliferation of stenting in the interventional community. A registry of 50 cases of rotational atherectomy in restenotic stents has demonstrated greater than 99% procedural success and a restenosis rate of 35%.[59] This recurrent restenosis rate is lower than reported for balloon treatment of in-stent restenosis. The clinical trial will be a three-arm randomization-PTCA vs. rotational atherectomy with or without low-pressure balloon angioplasty vs. rotational atherectomy followed by conventional adjunctive PTCA at standard pressure.

CARAT (Coronary Angioplasty and Rotational Atherectomy Trial)
CARAT is a prospective multicenter randomized trial which compares the results of Rotablator using small burrs (final burr-to-artery ratio < 0.7) versus large burrs (final burr-to-artery ratio > 0.7). The primary endpoint is final diameter stenosis; secondary endpoints include target lesion revascularization and cost. The study will enroll approximately 600 patients.

Summary
The accumulated clinical data demonstrates the safety and efficacy of the Rotablator system. Further studies applying refined techniques and the use of device synergy or pharmacological adjuvants will provide further clarification as to the optimal utilization for rotational atherectomy.

Procedure

Chapter 3

This chapter focuses on the procedural aspects of patients undergoing rotational atherectomy. The goal is a seamless guide for patient selection and management in the cardiac catheterization laboratory primarily directed towards Rotablator system issues which include decisions for guide catheters, guidewires, burr selection and adjunctive devices. Technique and strategy is fully described with pertinent examples, as well as the post-procedure management.

Patient Selection

Patient selection for the Rotablator system includes antecedent factors such as clinical status (stable vs. unstable angina), lesion characteristics, patency of remaining vessels, distribution of collateral flow and left ventricular function. Since the Rotablator not only impacts the lesion, but can affect the entire vessel (diffuse spasm or slow flow), and subsequently left ventricular function, the potential for deleterious effects can be increased if proper judgment is not applied to patient selection.

Clinical Status

The clinical presentation of the patient may have important implications as to the nature of the lesion to be treated, the status of the myocardium subtended by the vessel and the left ventricular function. Specifically, patients identified with unstable angina, myocardial infarction or post-infarction angina may have thrombus containing lesions that are less than optimally treated with rotational atherectomy. Patients with congestive heart failure or documented low ejection fractions present a greater challenge with rotational atherectomy due to the potential of associated transient left ventricular dysfunction.

The majority of patients have angina due to flow limiting obstructions that are predominantly stable plaques. If lesion morphology is undetermined and there are suggestions of a thrombus containing lesion, treatment with heparin for several extra days may be justified. Recently the use of ReoPro has shown promising results.

Lesion Morphology and Location

The impetus for an interventional cardiologist to select an alternative device to the standard of PTCA is to improve acute results and/or reduce restenosis. Restenosis rates for rotational atherectomy have yet to be defined and thus the major indication is to improve procedural outcome and to expand the indications of percutaneous revascularization. Therefore, despite the device being applicable to a broad spectrum of lesions, with the exception of thrombotic lesions and those in the body of saphenous vein grafts (soft elastic substrate), the device has often been "niched" into complex morphologies. These "signature" lesions have included those with significant calcification and those vessels with diffuse disease. Many of the lesions treated with rotational atherectomy could not to be crossed with a balloon or if the balloon was positioned at the lesion site were undilatable. The aorto-ostial (this is not an FDA approved indication) location, branch ostial, protected left main and the anastomosis junction between the saphenous vein graft and native vessel have lower success with PTCA and have been favored sites for rotational atherectomy. The next chapters will give a detailed analysis of the approach to both simple and complex lesions with the Rotablator system.

Patency of Untreated Vessels

Since rotational atherectomy can be associated with transient left ventricular dysfunction, the status of the remaining vessels is an important factor in assessing risk. Multivessel disease, should be considered a higher risk application for rotational atherectomy when compared to PTCA or stenting. Retrospective analysis of the multicenter registry revealed a higher incidence of major complications when treating the left coronary circulation in the presence of an occluded RCA.[60] Patients with multivessel disease should be treated with rotational atherectomy only by operators who have adequate experience with the device.

Left Ventricular Function

Left ventricular function needs to be documented prior to performing rotational atherectomy. For those patients with low ejection fractions, prophylactic placement of an intra-aortic balloon pump should be considered.[61] Inexperienced operators should avoid patients with poor left ventricular function, since even minimal pertubation in technique or judgment may result in higher complication rates.

Patient Selection Summary

In summary, when considering the Rotablator system, patient selection requires integration of clinical presentation, lesion characteristics, left ventricular function, and the patency of the untreated vessels. A comprehensive evaluation must be made of the potential effects of attenuated coronary flow on the patient's overall hemodynamics. The essential lesson from the multicenter registry includes thorough preprocedure evaluation to maximize optimal outcomes. There is a significant learning curve with the Rotablator System which needs to be respected.

Preprocedural Management

The preintervention management of patients undergoing rotational atherectomy is similar to that of other percutaneous devices with several caveats.

Premedication includes aspirin (325 mg orally) and calcium channel blockers. Calcium channel blockers, rather than beta blockers, are recommended. Calcium channel blockers may reduce the frequency of vasospasm, which occurs in approximately 15% of cases.

Adequate hydration plays an integral role for this procedure since the patients often receive generous amounts of vasodilators, predominantly nitroglycerin but also calcium channel blockers. The use of pulmonary artery catheters to assess filling pressures is generally reserved for cases with significantly compromised left ventricular function. In most cases, hypovolemia can be easily treated using the venous sheath sidearm port to infuse fluids. The insertion of a prophylactic intra-aortic balloon pump is considered in patients with complex lesions (e.g. heavily calcified, > 20 mm with a small distal bed) and severe left ventricular dysfunction, or in cases where the target vessel has a complex lesion and supplies the majority of the overall viable myocardium.[61]

The recent addition of vasodilators in the infusate that cools the Rotablator system and exits via the distal sheath has reduced the need for bolus injections and intravenous use. This subselective method of drug delivery is infused at a rate of approximately 7 cc/min. with the device inactivated (not spinning) and 13 cc/min. when the device is activated. The typical "cocktail" or "Rotaflush" has various concentrations and combinations of nitroglycerin, verapamil or heparin.[62,63] ReoPro preprocedure is presently being evaluated to potentially reduce slow flow and no reflow and subsequent CK elevation specifically in complex lesions.

The patients should be well sedated prior to the procedure, since they may have chest discomfort during the ablation and for several minutes afterward.

Vascular Access

Peripheral sheath size is determined by the guiding catheter required. The inner diameter of the guiding catheter should be 0.004" greater than the largest burr used during the procedure. Most large lumen 8 Fr guiding catheters will permit passage of up to a 2.15 mm burr; a large lumen 9 Fr catheter accommodates burrs up to 2.38 mm; a 10 Fr is required for the 2.50 mm burr (see Appendix, "Coronary Rotablator System Burr Size", page 286).

In addition to the arterial sheath, an 8 Fr venous sheath (oversized) is placed. The venous sheath is used as access for a temporary pacing wire or pressure monitoring catheters when warranted. In addition, the venous sheath sidearm provides a dedicated line for the liberal and rapid infusion of fluids when needed and is used to obtain venous blood for activated clotting times.

In the subset of high-risk patients in which an intra-aortic balloon pump may be urgently needed, an additional 6 Fr or 7 Fr arterial "prophylactic" sheath is recommended on the contralateral side for immediate access.

Temporary Pacemaker

Temporary pacemakers are used when treating vessels associated with the highest frequency of bradyarrhythmias and complete heart block. They include the right coronary artery and the dominant left circumflex. Occasionally heart block can be seen in treatment of the ostial LAD and when using large burrs ($\geq$ 2.25 mm). The slowing can occur anytime during the ablation but generally occurs with longer run times. The heart rate and baseline rhythm typically return shortly after the device is deactivated.

The mechanism of bradyarrythmias and heart block during rotational atherectomy is unclear. One theory suggests that it may be the result of microparticulate material embolizing to conductive sensitive tissue. Another theory suggests the trigger of some yet-to-be-described reflex. Interestingly, the onset of atrioventricular block has been occasionally observed while activating the device in the guiding catheter implying that microparticulate debris may not be the culprit.

Generally, the placement of the temporary pacemaker should be performed prior to heparinization to reduce the incidence of adverse sequelae in the rare event of a right ventricular perforation. The thresholds for capture should be ascertained as well as the hemodynamics during pacing. Low arterial pressures during pacing may indirectly indicate hypovolemia. Since diastolic blood pressure and, consequently, coronary blood flow is reduced during pacing, particulate clearance may be diminished and ablation times should be reduced once pacing has commenced.

The pacemaker is generally set at a rate of 50 beats per minute. If pacing continues after the device is deactivated, dialing down the rate until the intrinsic rhythm is reestablished is recommended to allow for the benefits of atrioventricular synchrony.

Catheters that provide both pacing and pressure monitoring capabilities have recently gained acceptance in a number of centers. Although pacemaker capture is generally less secure with these catheter electrodes, the benefit of pressure monitoring for these operators outweighs the disadvantage.

If pacemaker capture is lost during the procedure, immediately deactivating the Rotablator burr will generally reestablish the baseline rhythm. In the event that the rate does not return after deactivation of the device and the pacemaker has lost capture, asking the patient to cough has been shown to return the patient to baseline rhythm.

Intraprocedural Medication

Anticoagulation for Rotablator procedures follows similar guidelines to those of conventional PTCA. Additional vasodilators and analgesics may be required.

Although the frequency of severe vasospasm seems to be decreasing with recent technique modifications, and the use of a "Rotaflush", vasodilators may be required during the procedure. The most common method is to give a small bolus typically 100–150 µg of nitroglycerin. Smaller doses may accomplish the same or greater effect with a less significant impact on hemodynamics when given subselectively through a balloon or infusion catheter. In addition to nitroglycerin, verapamil and adenosine are being tested for their ability to treat vasospasm.

Vasopressors should be available during Rotablator procedures and the catheterization laboratory personnel should be experienced with the dose and administration. Vasopressors such as dopamine should be readily accessible and implemented in cases of hemodynamic compromise. In addition, some labs have neosynephrine, aramine and epinephrine available.

Finally, the use of analgesics is common during the procedure. Shortly after rotational atherectomy some patients have moderate to severe chest discomfort that requires attention. The combination of valium with medications such as morphine and fentanyl has provided effective levels of patient comfort.

Glycoprotein IIb/IIIa inhibitors such as ReoPro have gained acceptance based on data from the Epic and Epilog trials. Several experienced Rotablator operators have begun using ReoPro in the more complex cases and the initial "snapshot" indicates a lower incidence in flow attenuation during the procedure. The suggestion that slow flow or no reflow is a platelet mediated event has always been a consideration. The reduced incidence of CK elevation with rotational atherectomy and ReoPro supports this concept.[56] Further elucidation of the benefits of this class of compounds is the subject of a clinical trial (see Chapter 2, page 33).

"Rotaflush"*

- The addition of vasodilators to the flush bag. Typically, nitroglycerin and heparin with or without calcium channel blockers such as verapamil.

* Rotaflush is not FDA approved.

Guide Catheter Selection

Guide catheter selection is extremely important when performing rotational atherectomy. In most interventional procedures with other device modalities, the primary function of the guiding catheter is to provide a conduit to deliver the device to the designated segment. In Rotablator procedures, the guide catheter acts as the delivery system for the burr and has several additional influences. The guide catheter will determine the ease of advancement of the burr and the trajectory of the guidewire which orients the burr and affects the direction of the ablation plane.

Coaxial guide catheter alignment will reduce the tension or pull required on the guidewire when advancing the burr. Significant support or deep intubation generally is not needed with this device since activation of the burr provides orthogonal displacement of friction, which will reduce drag to ease the passage of the burr through the vessel (see page 82, "Methods of Burr Advancement").

Figure 3.1

Coaxial Guide Catheter Alignment

An Amplatz (AL2) produces an optimal trajectory for the burr to engage the lesion at the ostium of the ramus artery (arrow).

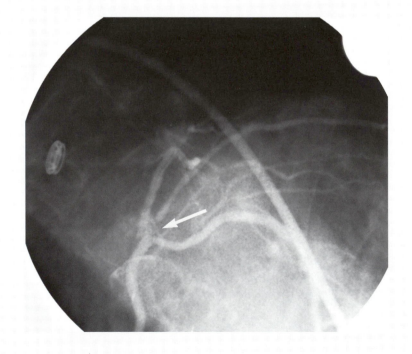

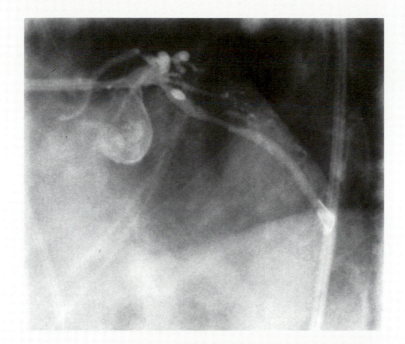

Figure 3.2 A&B

Eccentric Burr Trajectory

A) The guide catheter and/or the left main can direct the guidewire and the burr eccentrically with a tangential trajectory.

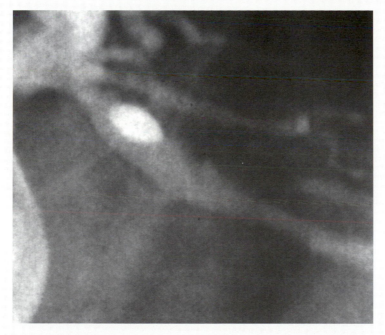

B) This enlarged view of the Rotablator burr shows its asymmetric orientation within the vessel. If activated, the burr would preferentially ablate the superior surface of the vessel.

Figure 3.3

Eccentric Burr Trajectory

The skewed trajectory of the burr is determined by the guide catheter position.

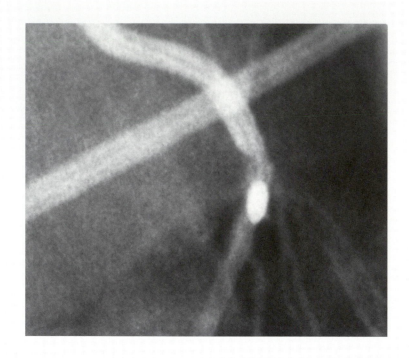

Coaxial Alignment
- Prevents tangential cutting
- Eases burr advancement
- Facilitates coaxial guidewire placement

A more subtle and consequential issue in guide selection is the manner in which it orients the guidewire (Figures 3.1, 3.2 and 3.3). As can be seen in Figure 3.4, guide catheters with similar designations (both JL-4) from different manufacturers may have distinctively different orientation in the vessel based on the differences in the primary and secondary curves. In Figure 3.4A, the burr would be oriented to the superior surface of the vessel. The optimal guide catheter should be coaxial (Figure 3.4B) to orient the guidewire centrally, therefore avoiding guidewire bias. An example is the use of an Amplatz shape in the treatment of an ostial circumflex lesion. Amplatz guides can often be manipulated to "telescope" into the circumflex resulting in a centrally positioned guidewire. Judkins curves that are generally not directed toward the circumflex would cause the burr to cut primarily on the inner curve of the ostial circumflex lesion, (i.e. the wall contiguous with the left main).

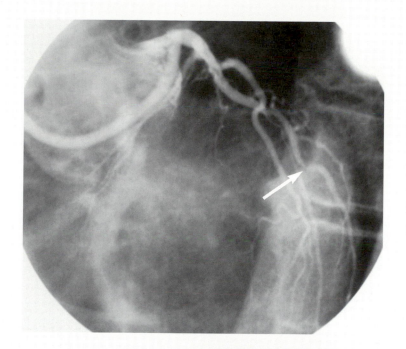

Figure 3.4 A&B

Guide Catheter Selection

A) (A) and (B) represent JL-4 guide catheters from two different manufacturers in the same left main coronary artery. The superior orientation of the guide catheter in (A), would make advancement of the burr difficult and would create a tangential ablation vector. Therefore, this guide catheter was exchanged for a JL-4 with a less pronounced curve. The lesion is distal at the bifurcation (arrow).

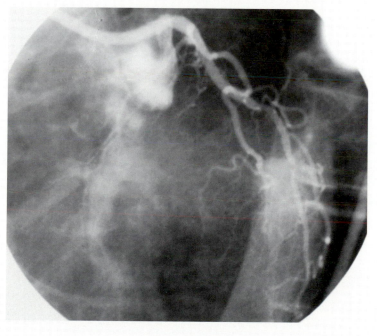

B) The new guide catheter provided better coaxial alignment for rotational atherectomy, easing burr advancement and reducing guidewire bias.

The concept of the "active" guide catheter can be applied during rotational atherectomy. In cases where an eccentric lesion is treated, the guide catheter can be manipulated to permit the guidewire to orient closer to the lesion, such that the advancing burr can achieve improved engagement or "purchase" of the lesion. This concept is referred to as "directional" rotational atherectomy. By manipulating the guide catheter, the burr, via the guidewire, is directed toward the lesion. One would expect in these cases to achieve a lumen larger than the size of the burr selected.[7]

The guide catheter inner diameter should be .004" larger than the largest burr used. The vast majority of cases can be performed with a 9 Fr catheter (able to accommodate up to a 2.38 mm burr. See Appendix, page 286). In lesions such as ostial right coronary arteries (these are not an approved indication) rotating in the guide catheter may be necessary but should be limited to cases where the alignment is coaxial with the lesion. Therefore, oversizing the guide catheter may be helpful even for cases in which use of larger burrs is not anticipated. Larger guide catheters will limit the contact between the burr and the inner surface of the guide catheter. Firm guide catheter tips may also be beneficial since occasionally a soft tip guide catheter can "fish mouth" and hinder advancement of the large burrs.

Sideholes are recommended, since they will provide increased perfusion that can promote particle clearance throughout the procedure. The sideholes can also be used for hand injections of blood (manual balloon pump). This technique is discussed as a method to manage slow flow in Chapter 7, page 247.

The guide catheter is the foundation for the procedure. It determines how well the burrs advance (particularly the larger ones), and how the guidewire vectors in the vessel. These factors will ultimately impact the effectiveness of the treatment.

Guidewire Selection and Placement

As described in earlier sections and in the Appendix, (pages 270–271) there are several different guidewires available for the Rotablator system. The Type C, which has historically been the workhorse guidewire, is a 325 cm, 0.009" diameter stainless steel monofilament with a 3.7 cm platinum tip (Figure 3.5). The Type A guidewire has a similar shaft construction but with a shorter distal platinum tip (2.6 cm) and a core extending to the distal end making it stiffer and similar to a "standard" PTCA guidewire. The RotaWire Floppy is a guidewire recently designed that addresses some of the limitations of the Type C and the Type A. The RotaWire Floppy has a stainless steel transitional shaft that tapers from a 0.009" to 0.005" at the distal end with a 2.2 cm platinum tip (Figure 3.6). The transition provides the guidewire with greater torque, flexibility and tracking. The flexibility of the RotaWire Floppy in negotiating complex vessels is an obvious advantage; the ability to track the burr to the lesion and the impact on lesion ablation is being assessed.

The distal tip can be gently curved by the operator simply by compressing the bent tip between the thumb and forefinger. A

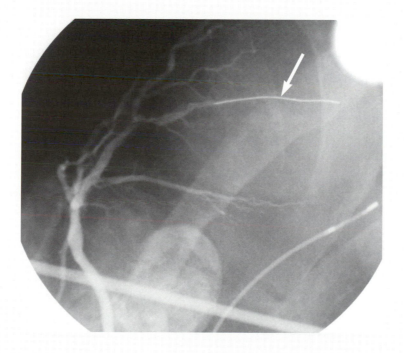

Figure 3.5

Type C Guidewire

The 3.7 cm radiopaque tip of the Type C guidewire (arrow) is clearly visible in the distal LAD. The potential limitation of this long distal tip in vessels with a short distal bed is apparent, since the burr cannot be advanced over this segment.

Figure 3.6

RotaWire Floppy Guidewire

The shorter 2.2 cm distal tip of the RotaWire Floppy guidewire (arrow) is seen here. Note in this angiogram the relatively proximal placement of the guidewire compared to conventional angioplasty technique. This more proximal placement will reduce axial stress of the guidewire and provide greater degrees of freedom for orientation of the burr. (See Figure 3.10).

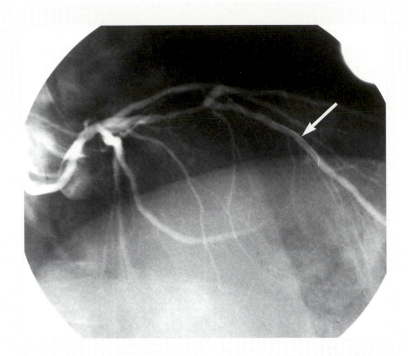

Small Branch Management

Contrast should flow freely around and beyond the distal tip to insure the guidewire is not in a small branch.

"ribboning technique" can stretch the platinum spring and should be performed carefully. The bare guidewire is inserted into an introducer sheath (to minimize blood loss and the possibility of kinking), advanced to the ostium of the vessel and then manipulated across the lesion and positioned in a distal segment. It helps significantly to remove the guidewire from the packaging loop and maintain it straight on the table. This technique will increase the torque performance of the guidewire. Rotating the guidewire between the fingers (similar to rolling a cigarette) while advancing can improve the tracking of the device (reduces sideload friction). The platinum tip must be distal to the lesion since the burr cannot track over this larger segment of guidewire. The tip should not be placed in a diminutive branch. Generally, the branch should be large enough so that contrast media can be demonstrated flowing past the tip. Occasionally in cases where the vessel has limited length beyond the lesion, guidewires with the shorter distal

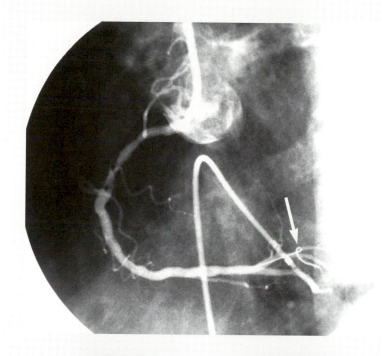

Figure 3.7 A&B

Guidewire Perforation

Case Information:
- Guide Catheter: 9 Fr Hockey Stick
- Guidewire: Type C
- Pacemaker: Yes
- Burrs: 1.75 mm, 2.25 mm
- PTCA: 4.5 x 20 mm

A) This case illustrates two aspects to avoid with the Rotablator guidewire (1) allowing the guidewire to loop, and (2) placement into a small distal branch (arrow).

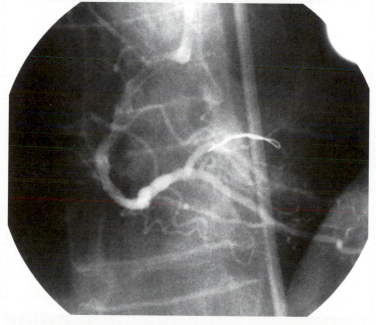

B) After completing the treatment of the proximal RCA lesion with a 4.5 mm balloon, the guidewire required significant force to be removed from the vessel due to the looped distal tip embedded in the vessel wall. A perforation resulted during withdrawal. There was minimal extravasation and no further therapy was required, since the site sealed spontaneously.

tips can be beneficial. Attempts should be made to keep the guidewire from prolapsing or coiling, since any rotation during burr activation can result in a fracture or a trapping of the tip in the vessel wall (Figure 3.7), especially in smaller branches.

When the Rotablator System guidewire cannot cross the lesion, the best strategy is to place a conventional guidewire and exchange for the Rotablator guidewire. Almost all balloon and transfer catheters with 0.014" lumens will have tolerance to accept the 0.009" guidewire for an exchange procedure. Experienced users rarely fail with the 0.009" Rotablator guidewire, because lesions that are difficult to cross due to observed tortuosity or rigidity can be recognized preprocedure. In tortuous or very rigid vessels the Type C and Extra Support guidewires conform poorly to the central lumen with high sideload forces directed toward the artery wall, making advancement difficult. The RotaWire Floppy is designed to address this problem with improved tracking and torquing.

Guidewire Positioning and Guidewire Bias

In rotational atherectomy the guidewire plays a paramount role in establishing the cutting vector of the device and therefore the position is crucial to the outcome of the procedure. The goal is to set the optimal ablation vector for treatment of the lesion while minimizing sideload forces at the segments proximal and distal to the lesion site. There exists a balance between the vessel and the guidewire in which the guidewire attempts to remain straight (its lowest energy state) and the vessel attempts to remain in its natural configuration. When the guidewire has greater rigidity than the vessel, pseudolesions occur and the vessel is deformed from the native architecture (Figures 3.12 and 3.13). When the vessel is more rigid than the guidewire, the guidewire yields to the configuration of the artery and places tension on the wall at points of contact. This tension may make burr advancement more difficult (Figure 3.8) and may affect ablation. Therefore, once the guidewire is in place, an angiogram is performed to assess the interaction between the guidewire and the vessel. Often in a vessel with

Guidewire Bias

The tangential trajectory of the guidewire from the central axis of the vessel may be due to:

- Guide catheter orientation
- Vessel architecture: tortuous, angulated or branching
- Vessel compliance: elastic vs. inelastic

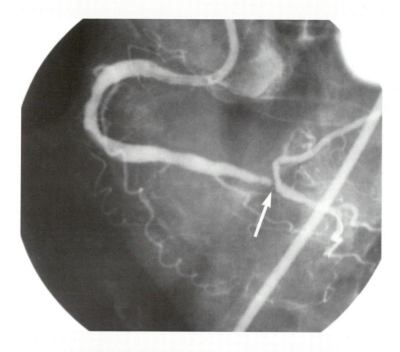

Figure 3.8 A&B

Guidewire/Burr Interaction in a Rigid Vessel

Case Information:
- Guide Catheter: 8 Fr Hockeystick
- Guidewire: Type C
- Pacemaker: Yes
- Burrs: 1.5 mm
- PTCA: 3.5 x 20 mm @ 3 atm

A) In this 83 year-old female the RCA was large, severely calcified and inelastic. The balance between the guidewire and the vessel favored the vessel and resulted in the guidewire straining against the rigid wall. A small 1.5 mm burr was unable to be advanced nonactivated beyond the ostium. Low-speed advancement (120,000 rpm) was required to position the burr in the distal segment (arrow).

B) Post-atherectomy, a 3.5 mm balloon at 3 atm achieved this final result.

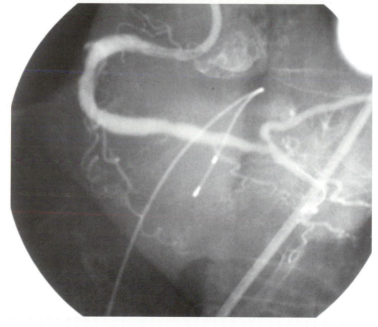

Balance of Force in Vessels

Elastic Vessels: The guidewire in an elastic vessel favors the tensile strength of the guidewire, and the vessel distorts (creating pseudolesions or wrinkling). The tension from the guidewire on the artery may exceed the elasticity of the vessel and result in cutting.

Inelastic Vessels: In inelastic vessels the guidewire bends or curves with the vessel and usually lies preferentially to one side.

tortuosity beyond the lesion, the distal vector forces may change the orientation of the guidewire at the lesion producing preferential cutting to one wall. If there is tension from the guidewire on the wall, preferential cutting can be further amplified (Figure 3.9). Retracting the guidewire to a proximal position (Figure 3.10), may improve coaxial alignment at the lesion site. The guidewire should also be retracted to a more proximal position if pseudolesions are prominent distally. Deformity of the artery due to the guidewire in the segment proximal to the lesion will impact the vector of the burr as it approaches the lesion and will often limit the burr sizes that can be used (Figure 3.12). The proximal deformity or pseudolesions may result in ablation of normal tissue if the strain on the wall by the guidewire is excessive.

From the above discussion, it is evident that the guidewire position in the artery is a major determinant for optimal treatment. Only rarely are the guide catheters ideally coaxial and the vessels straight (Figure 3.11). More often the vessels are angulated and tortuous and the guidewire will have a tendency to project out of the central axis of the vessel. The divergence from the central axis of the vessel is referred to as guidewire bias. Guidewire bias may be unfavorable when it orients the burr out of the central plane of the vessel and, due to the tension on the artery, results in radial or tangential ablation[64] or, in extreme cases, perforation (see Chapter 7, page 254). In cases where the trajectory of the guidewire is directed away from a lesion, engagement of the plaque may be difficult and manipulation of the guidewire position, or guide catheter may be beneficial. Guidewire bias can be beneficial when it orients the burr toward the lesion (favorable guidewire bias) (Figure 3.15).[65] In cases with favorable guidewire bias, larger lumens can be achieved than the size of the burr and subsequent burr sizes should be predicated on these results, i.e. larger burrs may not be required.

Once the guidewire is positioned, a burr is selected and backloaded onto the guidewire and tested outside the body proximal to the O-ring. The burr is then advanced easily through

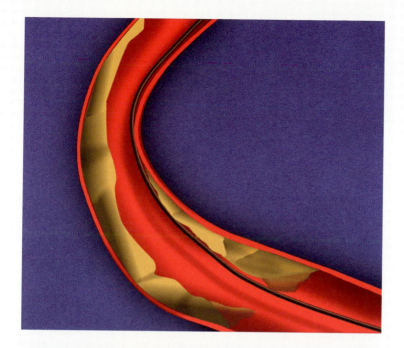

Figure 3.9 A&B

Preferential Cutting

A) The guidewire is shown preferentially oriented to the inner wall of the vessel.

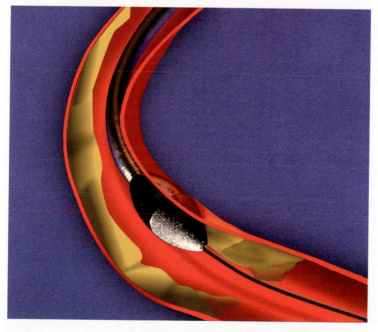

B) The burr follows the guidewire preferentially cutting along one wall of the vessel. If the tension of the guidewire exceeds the elastic threshold of the vessel, healthy tissue will be ablated.

Figure 3.10 A&B

Guidewire Axial Tension as Determined by Distal Placement

A) A guidewire that is placed distally can create a tethering effect, causing the burr to be oriented tangentially in a tortuous vessel. Because the burr will follow the course of the guidewire, it will be forced against one wall. While this may be advantageous when eccentric plaque is confined to the inner curvature of the vessel, plaque on the outer curve may not be treated.

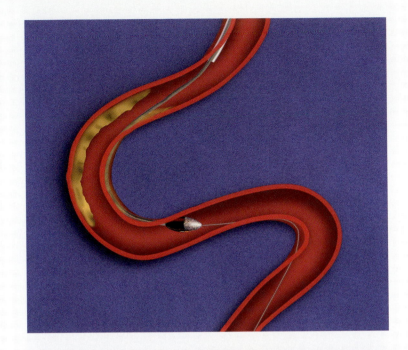

B) Positioning the guidewire just distal to the lesion can virtually eliminate the tethering effect. The increased guidewire freedom allows the burr to remain centered, resulting in concentric ablation of the lesion. Care must be taken to ensure that the spring tip of the guidewire is positioned beyond the lesion, as the burr cannot be advanced over this segment.

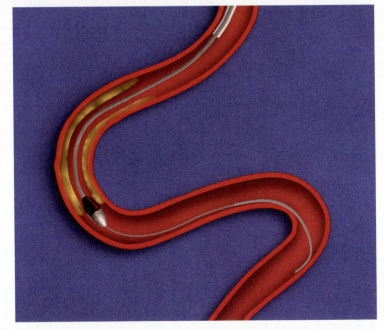

the guide catheter until it reaches the distal primary and secondary curves. In order to advance further, tension is required on the guidewire and, to deliver the burr into the artery, a tapping motion on the burr via the driveshaft will ease exiting from the guide catheter. Problems entering the artery are typically secondary to misalignment of the guide catheter with the ostium of the vessel. As the device negotiates the coronary artery, the burr may become more difficult to advance and greater tension on the guidewire may be required. Extreme amounts of tension applied to the system, especially in tortuous vessels can cause the guidewire to become taut (Figure 3.10), resulting in excessive force directed against the vessel wall. The lateralization of the guidewire onto the wall can result in ablation (Figure 3.14) if the burr is advanced in an activated mode. Therefore if the nonactivated burr is not advancing easily through the vessel, prior to converting to an activated advancement technique, relieve the tension on the guidewire. In cases where, with tension, the burr is successfully placed in the platform segment proximal to the lesion, it is prudent to release the tension on the system prior to treatment. The tension on the guidewire can be relieved by first relieving driveshaft tension as described on page 87. Then activate the device depressing the brake defeat button with the wireClip in place and minimally advance and withdraw the guidewire to confirm that there is "play" or the lowest possible tension in the system.

After advancing the burr to the platform segment just proximal to the lesion, reassess the lie of the guidewire and adjust if needed, relieve driveshaft tension as described on page 87 and inject contrast to assess the cutting vector of the burr.

Guidewire Case Studies and Graphic Illustrations

Rotational atherectomy does not lend itself to a simple formula, but rather, requires a continuous interrogation and updating as the case proceeds. In the following examples, strategies for burr selection and adjunctive therapies were modified due to subtle but important guidewire issues. (Text resumes on page 70.)

Checking for Guidewire Bias

Performing an angiogram after placement of the guidewire is critical to assess the guidewire-vessel interaction.

Figure 3.11 A&B

Preferred Guidewire Positioning

Case Information:
- Guide Catheter: 9 Fr JR-4
- Guidewire: Type C
- Pacemaker: Yes
- Burrs: 1.5, 2.0 mm
- PTCA: 3.5 mm x 30 mm @ 1.5 atm.

A) This 66 year-old male had minimal disease in the left coronary system and a heavily calcified 90% stenosis in the ostium of the RCA. The angiogram shows optimal positioning of the guide catheter and guidewire. The guide catheter is coaxial and the guidewire is placed in the mid segment creating a central trajectory.

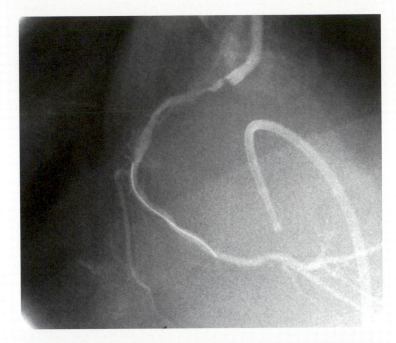

B) The burr is shown aligned properly for treatment. In aorto-ostial* lesions, platforming the burr in the guide catheter may be necessary, although not recommended. Therefore, larger guide catheters are used. (Final result not shown.)

Treatment of aorto-ostial lesions is not an FDA approved indication.

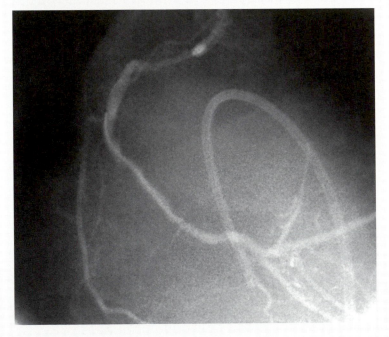

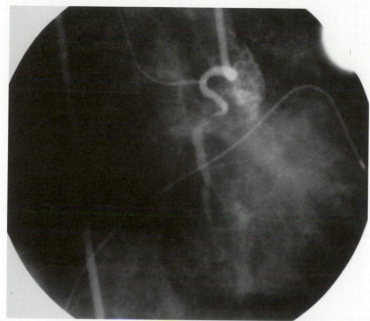

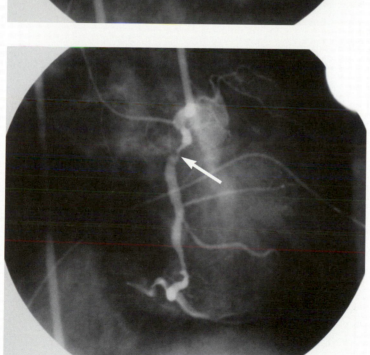

Figure 3.12 A-F

**Guidewire Effect on
Proximal Tortuosity**

Case Information:
- Guide Catheter: 8 Fr JR-4
- Guidewire: Type C
- Pacemaker: Yes
- Burrs: 1.25, 1.5 mm
- PTCA: 3.0 mm x 30 mm
  @ 3 atm.

A) This 58 year-old male with
a history of hypertension and
smoking was admitted for
elective angioplasty.
Angiography revealed a 90%
proximal and an 80% distal
stenosis of the RCA. The RAO
view prior to guidewire
insertion demonstrates the
marked proximal tortuosity of
the vessel.

B) After guidewire
placement, the vessel is
distorted. The highly angulated
lesion is straightened by the
guidewire (arrow) which will
change the cutting vector of
the burr.

Figure 3.12 C&D
continued

C) In the LAO view, the vessel appears much less tortuous. Pseudolesions were created by the tension of the stiff guidewire on the vessel wall (arrow).

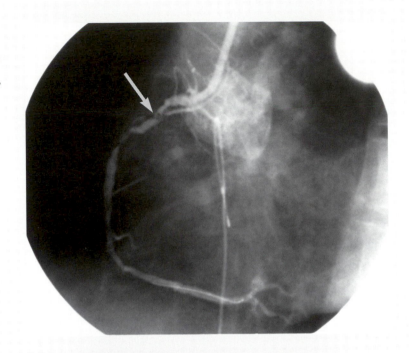

D) This LAO view shows the trajectory of the 1.25 mm burr. The vessel demonstrated pseudolesions proximal to the lesion due to the balance between a stiff Type C guidewire placed in a tortuous elastic vessel. Advancing the device nonactivated whenever possible is recommended to limit ablation of the wall in these segments.

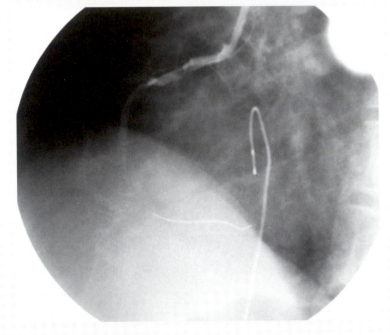

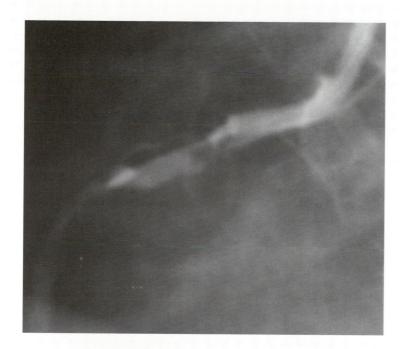

Figure 3.12 E&F
continued

E) The pseudolesions and the severe guidewire bias, are shown in this magnified view. Burrs were significantly undersized by 0.25–0.5 mm than would conventionally be used had this been a straight segment (final burr-to-artery ratio 0.6, see "Burr Selection" page 70). Vessels with proximal tortuosity or lesions on angulated segments mandate the use of undersized burrs and a strategy of lesion modification (page 97).

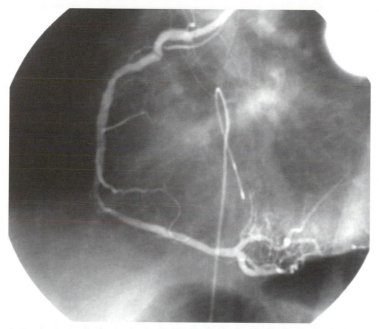

F) After treatment with 1.25 mm and 1.5 mm burrs, adjunctive PTCA was used rather than larger burrs due to the tortuosity and pseudolesions. A 3.0 x 30 mm balloon was inflated to 3 atm with this final result.

Figure 3.13 A-D

**Guidewire Effect on
Distal Tortuosity**

Case Information:
- Guide Catheter: 8 Fr JL-4
- Guidewire: Type C
- Pacemaker: No
- Burrs: 1.5, 1.75 mm
- PTCA: 2.5 x 20 mm
  @ 2 atm

A) In this LAO cranial view
prior to placement of the
guidewire, the LAD artery is
tortuous with an 80% stenosis
in the proximal vessel. The
lesion (arrow) is difficult to see
due to contrast blush in the
aortic root.

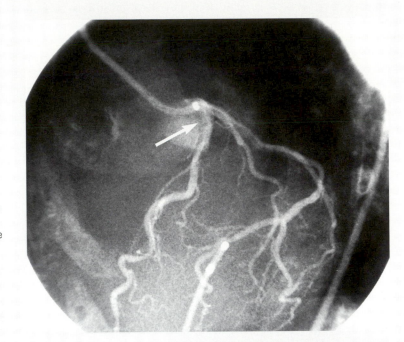

B) After guidewire placement,
numerous pseudolesions are
present in the distal vessel.
Since the lesion is proximal,
retracting the guidewire to
eliminate the pseudolesions
would not affect the ability
to treat the lesion (see
Figure 3.10).

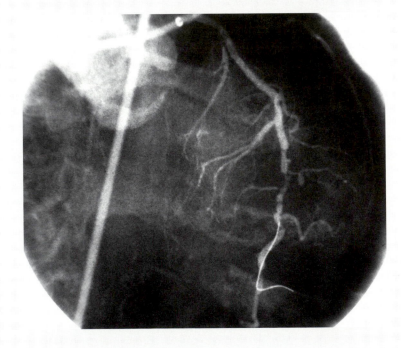

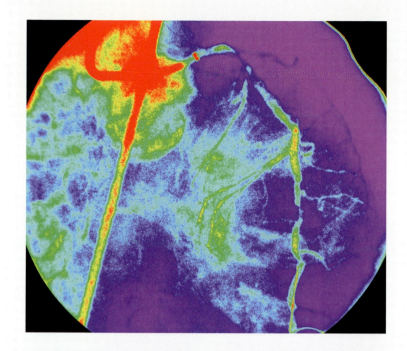

Figure 3.13 C&D
continued

C) False-color enhancement of (B) showing the pseudolesions caused by the guidewire.

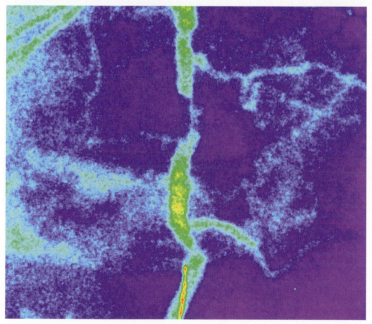

D) This false-color close-up shows the pseudolesions created by the guidewire in this vessel. The pressure of the guidewire causing vessel deformity may exceed the elasticity of the normal vessel, making it effectively inelastic and resulting in the removal of normal tissue if the burr is advanced into these segments.

Figure 3.14 A-D

Guidewire Bias Resulting in a Neolumen

Case Information:
- Guide Catheter: 8 Fr JL-4
- Guidewire: Type C
- Pacemaker: Yes
- Burrs: 1.5 mm
- PTCA: 1.5 x 30 mm
  @ 6 atm; 3.0 x 30 mm
  @ 3 atm.

A) This 58 year-old male with stable exertional angina was referred for rotational atherectomy after a failed PTCA secondary to an inability to cross the lesion. He had a 90% stenosis in the mid-LAD just beyond a severe bend followed by an 80% lesion in a heavily calcified vessel (arrows).

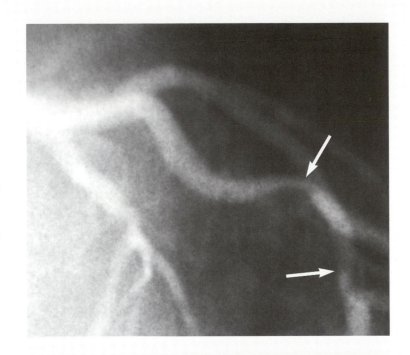

B) A nonactivated 1.5 mm burr could not be advanced to the lesion. Activating the device to advance the burr created a neolumen proximal to the lesion due to the upward force of the guidewire.

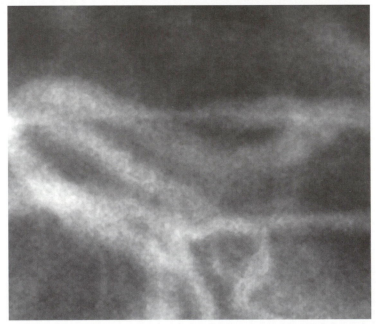

Figure 3.14 C&D
continued

C) This graphic interpretation shows the interaction of the burr, guidewire and vessel wall. Attempts to advance the nonactivated burr by pulling on the guidewire resulted in increased tension on the superior surface of the vessel. The burr "gutters" the vessel when activated.

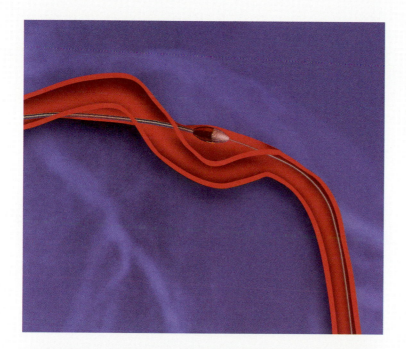

D) Activation of the device in the proximal LAD resulted in the neolumen in the curved segment of the vessel shown with the burr superimposed on the final result. TIMI III flow and 25% residual stenosis were present at the site of the lesions, and no further treatment was needed.

If the tension on the guidewire had been released prior to activation of the device, ablation of the wall may have been reduced. The RotaWire Floppy guidewire may also have been beneficial in this case.

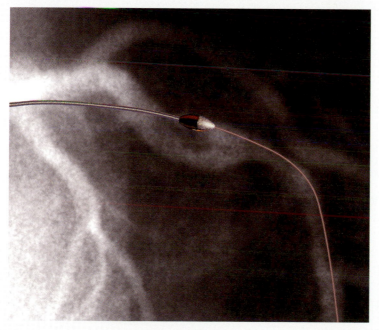

Figure 3.15 A-H

Favorable Guidewire Bias

Case Information:
- Guide Catheter: 9 Fr AL1
- Guidewire: Type C and Type A
- Pacemaker: Yes
- Burrs: 1.75 mm, 2.25 mm
- PTCA: 4.0 x 18 mm @ 5 atm

A) This 61 year-old man with previous bypass surgery presented with exertional angina and had two stenoses (arrows) in the left main coronary artery. The LAD was protected with a LIMA graft. The SVG to the dominant circumflex was occluded.

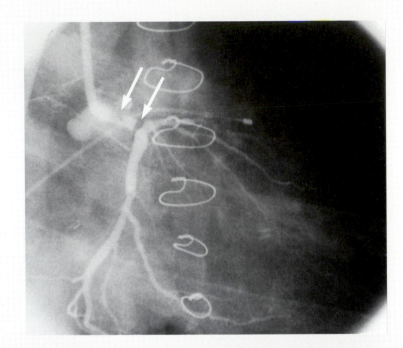

B) Rotational atherectomy was begun with the Type C guidewire in the circumflex and the 1.75 and 2.25 mm burrs. Post-atherectomy, significant stenoses remained due to the guidewire directing the cutting vector of the burrs away from the majority of plaque which was on the superior surface of the left main.

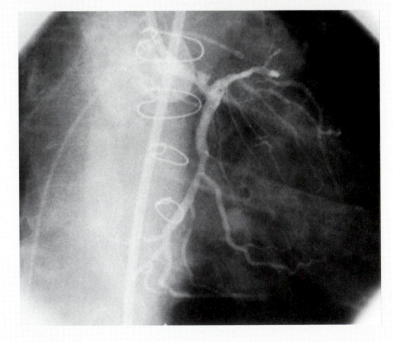

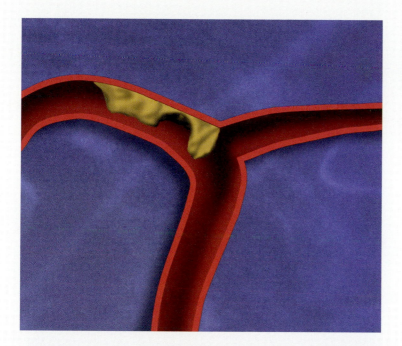

Figure 3.15 C&D
continued

C) In this graphic interpretation, the eccentric lesions on the superior surface of the left main are shown. The guidewire was initially placed in the circumflex artery (the compromised artery) since the LAD is protected by an internal mammary graft.

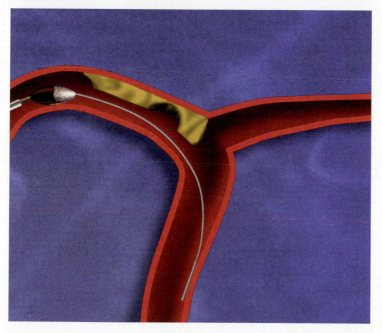

D) Significant plaque remained after atherectomy with the guidewire in the circumflex.

Figure 3.15 E&F
continued

E) The Type C wire was removed and replaced with a Type A wire in diagonal branch. The Type A wire was used because of a limited distal bed to place the platinum tip. With the guidewire in the diagonal, the 1.75 mm burr (arrow) was vectored directly into the lesion as shown demonstrating favorable guidewire bias. The lumen produced by the 1.75 mm burr was larger than predicted and additional burrs were not needed.

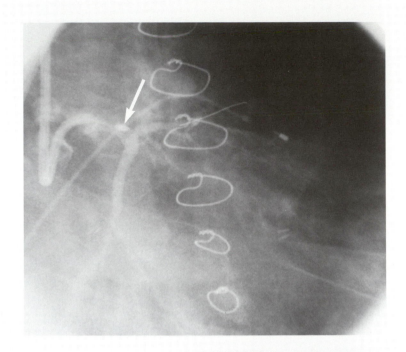

F) Post-atherectomy adjunctive PTCA was performed with a 4.0 mm balloon at 5 atm with this final result.

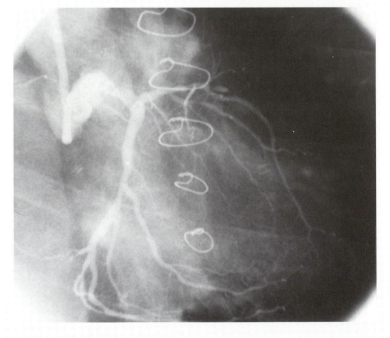

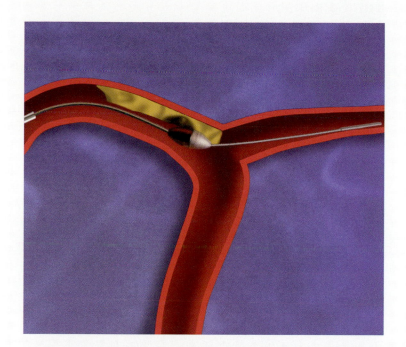

Figure 3.15 G&H
continued

G) The guidewire was repositioned into the LAD/Dx to improve the engagement of plaque with the burr demonstrating favorable guidewire bias.

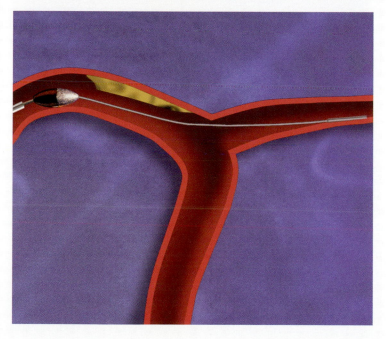

H) Graphic interpretation post-ablation. The favorable guidewire bias resulted in directional rotational atherectomy of the plaque.

Burr Selection

- Maximal burr is generally 60–85% of reference diameter
- Start with a burr 0.5 mm smaller than the largest anticipated burr
- Continuously modify decisions based on results after each burr pass

Burr Selection

Burr selection is predicated on a mosaic of interrelated parameters including vessel size, lesion morphology, distal vascular bed, segmental and global left ventricular function, and status of the remaining vessels. Some lesions benefit from a more aggressive approach of debulking, while others, due to anatomical features, are better managed with lower burr-to-artery ratios. Despite this heterogeneity several "rules" can be stipulated.

The conventional and most commonly used method for burr selection is as follows; assess the nominal vessel size, take 60–85% of that dimension as the maximal burr size to be used, and then reduce by 0.5 mm for the initial burr (Figure 3.16).

An example would be a vessel deemed to be 2.8 mm, approximately 75% is 2.1, therefore, the final burr would be between 2.25 mm (closer to 80%) or 2.0 mm (closer to 70%). The decision whether to use the 2.0, 2.15 or 2.25 mm burr would be

Figure 3.16 A-C

Conventional Burr Selection

Case Information:
- Guide Catheter: 8 Fr JL-4
- Guidewire: RotaWire Floppy
- Pacemaker: No
- Burrs: 1.5, 2.0 mm
- PTCA: 3.0 x 30 mm @ 2 atm

A) This 74 year-old woman had a myocardial infarction treated with TPA 5 days prior to this procedure. Subsequent angiography revealed diffuse disease in the LAD.

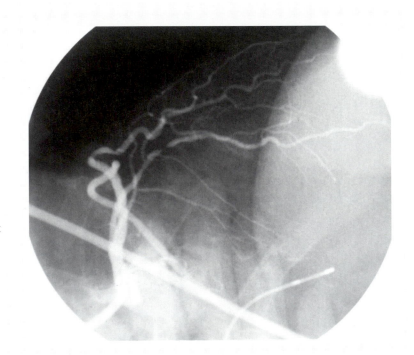

Figure 3.16 B&C
continued

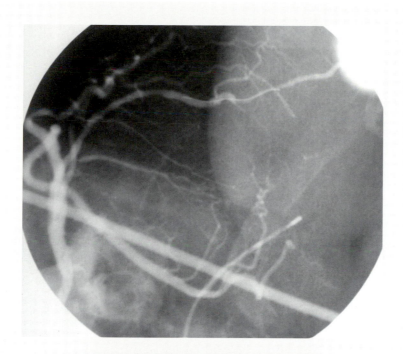

B) The reference vessel was estimated to be 2.5 mm. A final burr of 2.0 mm represents an 80% burr-to-artery ratio. The guide catheter is well aligned and the guidewire appears to be coaxial in the vessel. Therefore, an 80–85% burr-to-artery ratio is achievable. The procedure was therefore begun with a 1.5 mm burr followed by a 2.0 mm burr.

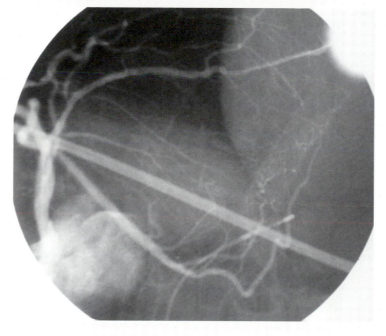

C) After atherectomy, treatment was completed with a 3.0 mm balloon at 2 atm.

based on overall vessel characteristics (can the device be safely delivered to the lesion), plaque burden, distal runoff, and left ventricular function. Elements that would support initiating, and possibly finishing with a smaller final burr are as follows:

- Proximal vessel characteristics such as tortuosity making it difficult to advance the device to the lesion (Figure 3.8 and 3.12)
- Lesion angulation greater than 60°
- Guidewire bias
- Excessive plaque burden (long lesions, heavily calcified lesions)
- Slow flow, severe chest pain, ECG changes, hemodynamic compromise with initial burr

Flexibility after analyzing the results after each burr is essential throughout the procedure to modify subsequent burr selection. Specific vessel and lesion subsets are presented the following chapters.

Burr Selection Case Studies

Burr selection remains one of the more difficult aspects for the Rotablator operator. It must take into account patient characteristics such as left ventricular function and hemodynamic stability, the vessel characteristics such as size, tortuosity and angulation, the lesion characteristics of length, calcification and potential plaque burden and the interaction of these characteristics with the device. Furthermore, it must be reevaluated continuously throughout the procedure.

The following five cases illustrate strategies for burr selection including some complex cases where the procedure was successful because burr selection was modified by intraprocedural variables and others where, in retrospect, the burr selection contributed to a poor outcome. What will be evident is that in a significant number of cases, burr selection does not lend itself to a simple formula. (Text resumes on page 82.)

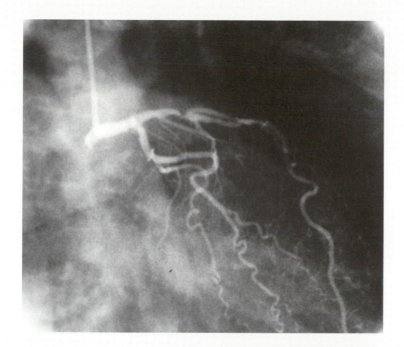

Figure 3.17 A&B
Standard Burr Selection

Case Information:
- Guide Catheter: 8 Fr JL-4
- Guidewire: Type C
- Pacemaker: No
- Burrs: 1.5, 2.0 mm
- PTCA: 3.0 x 30 mm
  @ 1 atm

A) A standard burr-selection strategy was used in this restenotic lesion in the LAD of a 76 year-old white female. The guidewire was placed just beyond the lesion to avoid distortion of the distal vessel. The vessel had a reference diameter of approximately 2.6 mm. A stepped-burr treatment was initiated with a 1.5 mm burr and completed with a 2.0 mm burr.

B) After treatment with 1.5 and 2.0 mm burrs and a 3.0 mm balloon at 1 atm, the lesion was reduced to a 10% residual stenosis.

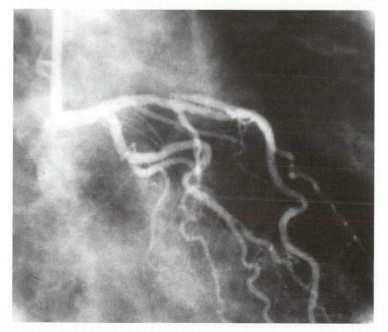

Figure 3.18 A-D

Burr Selection with Guidewire Bias

Case Information:
- Guide Catheter: 9 Fr JL-4.5
- Guidewire: RotaWire Support
- Pacemaker: No
- Burrs: 1.5, 2.0 mm
- PTCA: 3.5 x 30 mm @ 3 atm

A) This 71 year-old female had ostial and mid segment lesions in the LAD. IVUS revealed a 3.1 mm reference diameter just beyond the ostial lesion and a 2.9 mm diameter more distally.

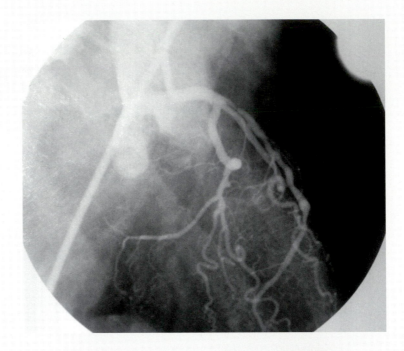

B) The LAD was treated from the ostium to the 90° bend using segmental ablation.

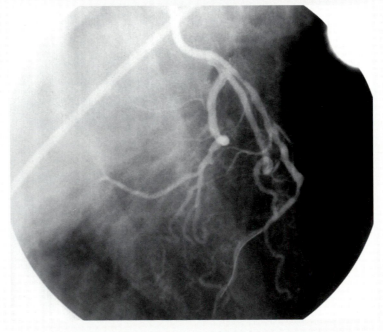

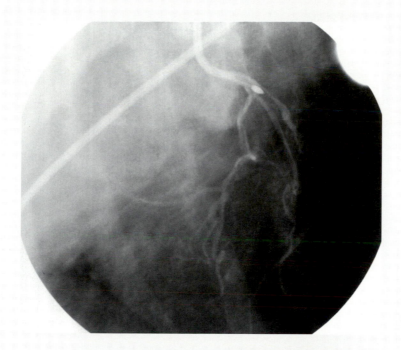

Figure 3.18 C&D
continued

C) A 2.0 mm burr, seen exiting from the guide catheter, demonstrated an inferior lie due to the trajectory provided from the guide catheter and guidewire. A larger burr was not used due to concerns of excessive ablation to the inferior wall of the vessel.

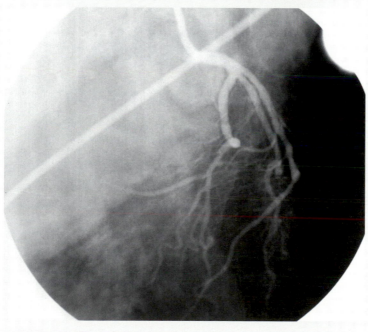

D) After atherectomy, treatment was completed with a 3.5 x 30 mm balloon.

Figure 3.19 A-D

Burr Selection in Total Occlusions

Case Information:
- Guide Catheter: 8 Fr JL-4
- Guidewire: Type C
- Pacemaker: No
- Burrs: 1.25, 1.5, 1.75 mm
- PTCA: 3.0 x 30 mm
  1–4 atm

A) This 59 year-old male, who presented 4 days earlier with a subendocardial infarction, was found to have a totally occluded LAD (arrow). After trying multiple guidewires, the lesion was finally crossed with a Silk™ wire (Cordis). A 2.0 mm balloon was inflated to 2 atm without evidence of balloon expansion due to heavy calcification at the site of occlusion.

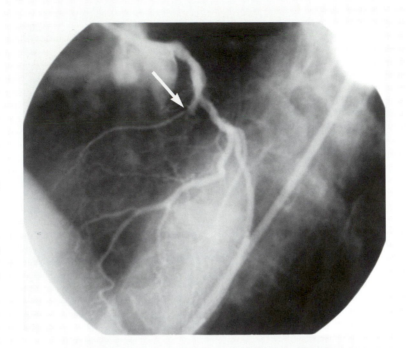

B) The Silk wire was exchanged through the balloon catheter for a Type C guidewire. A 1.25 mm burr was selected as the initial burr to achieve a "pilot channel".

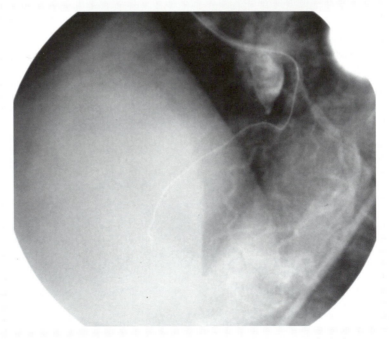

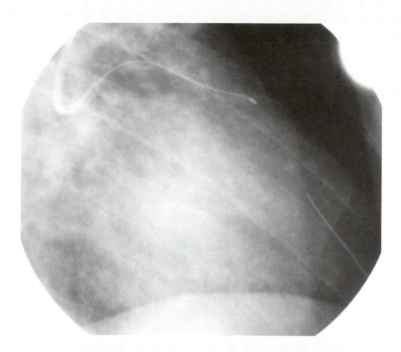

Figure 3.19 C&D
continued

C) The 1.25 mm burr was advanced smoothly through the total occlusion. Subsequent burrs of 1.5 and 1.75 mm were used. Small burr increments were used since the true lumen was poorly defined and the distal reference diameter was not known.

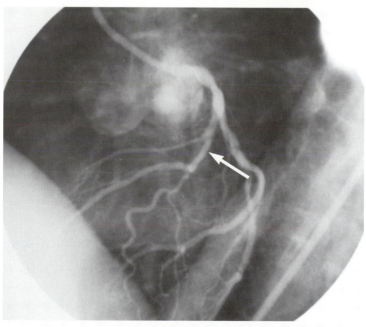

D) Post-atherectomy there was diffuse spasm in the distal LAD which was treated with a 3.0 mm balloon inflated at 1–2 atm and intracoronary nitroglycerin. The proximal area of heavy calcification was treated with a balloon inflated to 4 atm to achieve this final result (arrow).

Figure 3.20 A-D

Burr Selection in the Presence of Vessel Tortuosity

Case Information
- Guide Catheter: 8 Fr JL-4
- Guidewire: Type C
- Pacemaker: Yes
- Burrs: 1.5 mm
- PTCA: 2.5 x 2.0 mm @ 2 atm

A) This pretreatment angiogram shows an LAD lesion on a significant bend (arrow).

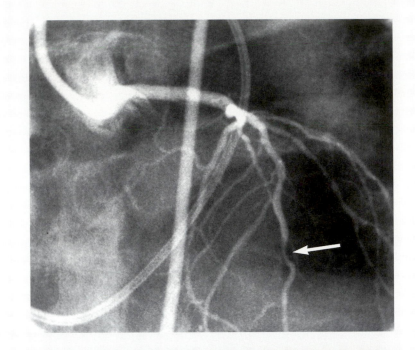

B) The Type C guidewire straightened the mid to distal LAD with guidewire bias favoring the superior aspect of the vessel. The platinum tip was advanced further prior to treatment.

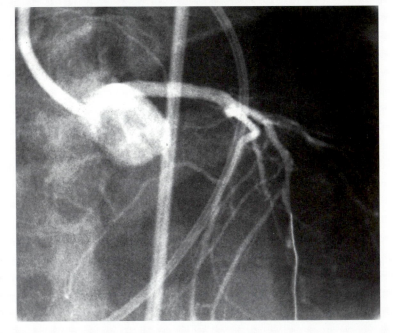

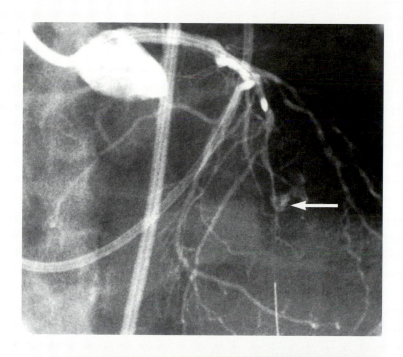

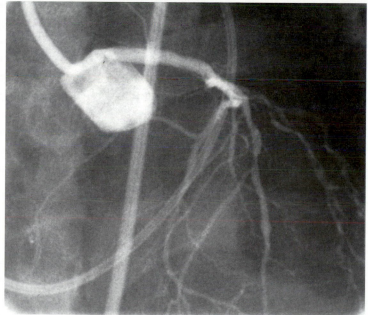

Figure 3.20 C&D
continued

C) A 1.5 mm burr resulted in a perforation at the lesion site (arrow). An angiogram after placing the guidewire can demonstrate guidewire bias and modify burr selection.

These lesions should be treated with undersized burrs. In this case a 1.25 mm burr may have been a more appropriate choice due to the vessel characteristics. In addition, releasing tension on the guidewire prior to ablation will maximize the potential for the burr to be centered. This can be accomplished by moving the guidewire forward and back to create "play" or decreased tension in the system. The RotaWire Floppy may be advantageous in these cases.

D) A prolonged inflation (15 minutes) with a 2.5 mm balloon sealed the perforation with this final result.

Figure 3.21 A&B

**Modified Burr Selection
with Suspected Thrombus**

Case Information:
- Guide Catheter: 9 Fr JL-4
- Guidewire: Type C
- Pacemaker: No
- Burrs: 1.75 mm
- PTCA: 3.0 x 20 mm
  @ 2–6 atm

A) This 62 year-old male presented with a restenotic lesion in the proximal LAD. Because it was a restenotic lesion, a larger burr (1.75 mm rather than 1.5 mm) was selected for the initial ablation. As a 2.25 mm burr was being advanced to the site, the patient developed an acute occlusion with chest pain and ECG changes. The 2.25 mm burr was removed without activation and replaced with a 3.0 mm perfusion balloon.

B) After 4 balloon inflations from 2–6 atm and intracoronary nitroglycerin, an excellent angiographic result was obtained and the patient's chest pain resolved. In the presence of chest pain and ECG changes, further Rotablator treatment should be withheld especially when the problem can not be solved with vasodilators or low-pressure PTCA. In this case thrombus was suspected due to the observed haziness of the lumen. The balloon was fully expanded at moderate pressures, implying a compliant lesion. Further incremental burrs were not required. Currently ReoPro would be considered in this situation.

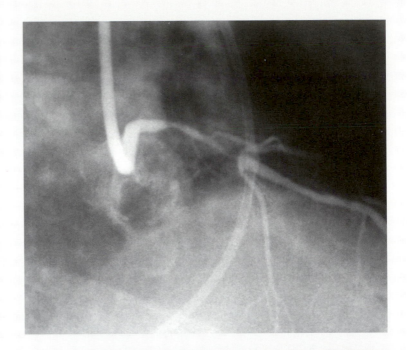

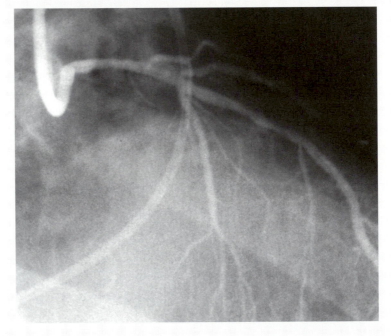

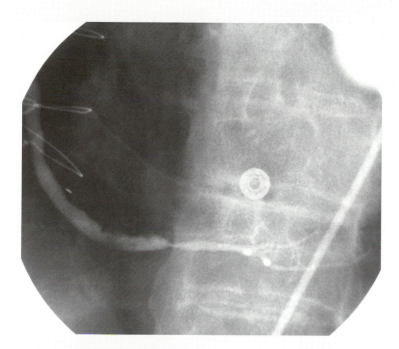

Figure 3.22 A&B

Inadequate Debulking

Case Information:
- Guide Catheter: Multipurpose
- Guidewire: Type C
- Pacemaker: Yes
- Burrs: 1.75 mm
- PTCA: 3.0 x 20 mm @ 12 atm

A) The lesion at the anastomosis of the saphenous vein graft to the RCA was treated with a 1.75 mm burr followed by a 3.0 mm balloon at 12 atm.

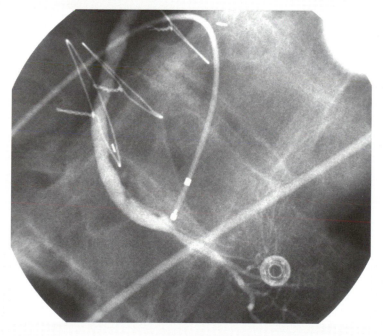

B) Post-procedure the lesion recoiled. Use of a larger burr to further increase compliance and lumen size may have been beneficial.

At the time of this procedure, atherectomy was not performed after balloon inflation. More recently, after balloon inflations up to 6 atm and no evidence of dissection, further atherectomy could be attempted (see "Interpolated Angioplasty", page 106).

High-Speed Test

Checklist (Outside the Body)

- Ensure that fluid is dripping from the distal sheath
- Verify competency of the brake
- Make sure advancer knob moves freely
- Verify burr speed
- Attach wireClip

Reasons for Failure to Achieve Target Burr Speed Outside the Body

- Kinked air hose
- Insufficient air pressure
- Kink in guidewire
- Lubrication removed from the guidewire or the guidewire is not properly cleaned or moistened.

High-Speed Test

After the burr is selected and the advancer has been connected to the console, the device is loaded onto the guidewire. The device should be advanced slowly over a clean, moistened guidewire to avoid accidental kinking. Advance the burr just proximal to the Y-connector. At this point the device is activated, it should be able to reach speeds between 180,000–190,000 rpm, depending on the burr size. In general, the outside speed should be approximately 10,000–20,000 rpm greater than what is desired in the platform segment proximal to the lesion. This is to accommodate the driveshaft having increased friction when over the guidewire. The curves of the guide catheter and coronary artery tortuosity increase the friction between the driveshaft and the guidewire resulting in reduced speed.

If the burr is unable to achieve the desired speed the most common causes include a kinked air hose, a kinked guidewire, insufficient air pressure or improper cleaning or moisturizing of the guidewire. These causes must be addressed before advancing the burr to the lesion.

In addition to assessing the speed, verify that fluid is exiting the Teflon sheath and check the competency of the brake by insuring that the guidewire with the burr activated is fixed.

Methods of Burr Advancement

Several methods have been advocated to advance the burr through the vessel to the treatment site. The following describes the technique options with respective advantages and disadvantages.

Nonactivated Burr Advancement

Nonactivated burr advancement is similar to advancing balloon catheters to the lesion site. The guidewire is braced in the artery with one operator applying a pulling force (tension) while the other operator advances the burr via the driveshaft. The burr can be easily advanced through the straight segments of the guide catheter. Resistance is initially felt as the burr approaches the primary and secondary curves of the distal tip of the guide catheter. By applying greater tension on the guidewire and a tapping motion to the burr via the driveshaft, the device will exit the guide catheter. Once in the artery, reaching the more distal aspects usually requires continued tension on the guidewire and further tapping on the driveshaft, until the burr can enter the platform segment.

The success of this burr advancement technique is largely dependent on the coaxial position of the guide catheter. The position is important to ensure that the tension on the guidewire is transmitted throughout the system. In most cases, this technique will be adequate to advance the burr to the platforming segment of the artery.

There are potential problems with this technique. In the event that significant force is required to "pull" or drag the burr into the vessel, this action can produce a taut guidewire or "drawstring" effect on the guidewire. This straightening of the guidewire may increase the sideload on the vessel and result in either a deformation of the vessel (pseudolesion) or an encroachment of the guidewire with tension against one of the vessel walls (Figures 3.12 and 3.13).

Activated Burr Advancement

There are two activated advancement techniques that can be performed to reach the lesion site. Low-speed advancement requires reducing the air turbine pressure and adjusting to approximately 100,000–120,000 rpm. This reduced speed will allow the burr to advance forward smoothly over the guidewire. Low-speed advancement will take advantage of orthogonal displacement of friction and ease the passage of the burr (Figure 3.8). Low-speed advancement is selected to minimize ablation of tissue in segments where the burr makes contact with tissue. By fixing the guidewire with the brake defeat engaged, the driveshaft is advanced forward gently (opposite of burr exchange). The use of Dynaglide is not recommended for advancement because the mechanism works on a servocontrol and if resistance is met, the console will automatically deliver more air pressure to retain the predesignated speed of 60,000 rpm. Therefore, the operator will not receive the feedback necessary for safe

Activated Advancement

The burr should not be activated unless contrast flows freely around it and driveshaft tension has been relieved. With the wireClip in place, depress the brake defeat, fix the guidewire and advance the system.

Low-Speed Advancement

- Speed 100,000– 120,000 rpm
- Not on Dynaglide

High-Speed Advancement

- Reserve for vessels with suspected occult narrowings
- Utilize the advancer knob for increased tactile feedback
- Speed > 140,000 rpm

advancement of the device.

High-speed advancement can also be utilized and should be reserved for those vessels where there may be occult narrowings not appreciated angiographically. Generally, with the high-speed technique, the burr is advanced with the advancer knob. By using high speed, the likelihood of ablation and plaque removal is greater as the device is advanced.

Prior to activating the device for advancement, tension needs to be relieved on the driveshaft or it may lurch forward upon activation. Follow the procedure described, "Relief of Driveshaft Tension", on page 87. In both activated advancement modes, prior to activating the burr, be certain the device is not in contact with the vessel by demonstrating unimpeded flow around the device.

In the rare situation when it is difficult to exit the burr from the guide catheter, it may be necessary to activate the device. Should activation be necessary, every effort should be made to attain the most favorable coaxial position between the guide catheter and ostium of the vessel.

Burr Advancement Case Study

The case in Figure 3.8 (page 53) demonstrated the classical use of low-speed advancement. Because of the guidewire tension against the wall of the large calcified RCA, a small 1.5 mm burr required low-speed advancement to reach the distal lesions site.

Figure 3.14 (page 64) demonstrated the formation of a neolumen which was created by high-speed advancement in the presence of a taut guidewire. Relief of guidewire tension is critical when significant force has been applied in an attempt to drag the burr to the lesion.

The following case study (Figure 3.23) illustrates unique problems associated with burr advancement. Generally difficulty with burr advancement involves distal lesions in vessels with proximal tortuosity or angiographically occult stenosis.

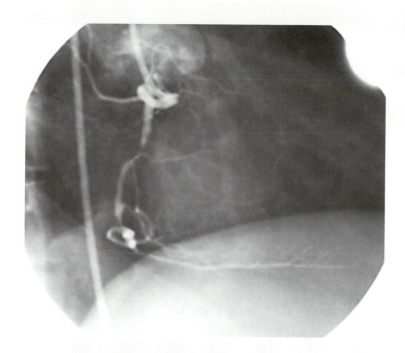

Figure 3.23 A-D

Burr Advancement in a Complex Vessel

Case Information:
- Guide Catheter: 8 Fr JR-4
- Guidewire: RotaWire Floppy, Type C
- Pacemaker: Yes
- Burrs: 1.5, 1.75, 2.0 mm
- PTCA: 3.0 x 30 mm @ 2 atm

A) This 52 year-old was found to have proximal and distal stenoses in a diffusely diseased and tortuous RCA.

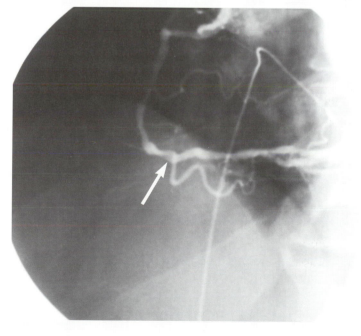

B) Because of the tortuosity of the artery, a RotaWire Floppy was used. The wire was inserted just beyond the distal lesion (arrow) to minimize sideload tension on the vessel, i.e. guidewire bias (see Figure 3.10).

Figure 3.23 C&D
continued

C) After treatment with the 1.5 mm burr, a 1.75 mm burr was selected but was unable to cross the tortuous segment in the distal vessel (arrow), even with activated advancement. The RotaWire Floppy was exchanged for the stiffer Type C wire and the burr was able to advance without difficulty.

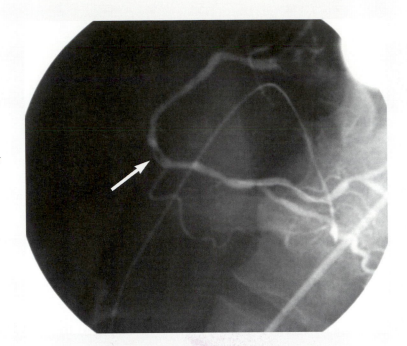

D) After the 1.75 mm burr, the proximal, mid and distal sites were treated with a 3.0 mm balloon at 4 atm with a significant residual stenosis remaining. The sites were then treated with a 2.0 mm burr followed by a 3.0 mm balloon at 4 atm with the result shown. (For a discussion of atherectomy after angioplasty, see "Interpolated Angioplasty", page 106).

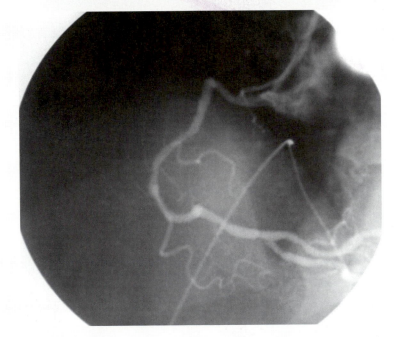

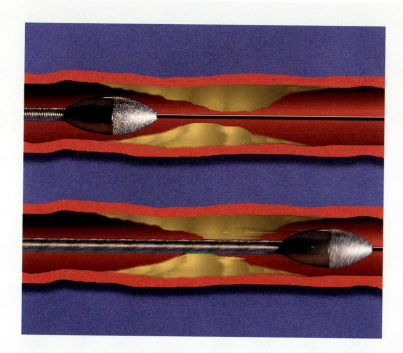

Figure 3.24

Driveshaft Compression

Driveshaft compression can develop as the burr is advanced into the platform segment. The driveshaft should be retracted at the Y-connector until the burr, visualized by fluoroscopy, begins to retract in the vessel.

Failure to decompress the driveshaft could cause the burr to lunge forward when activated (as shown in lower illustration).

Relief of Driveshaft Tension

As the burr is advanced to the platform segment, tension can develop in the driveshaft. The tension is a result of the compressibility of the driveshaft and is increased when it is difficult to advance the burr to the platform segment. To relieve the tension on the driveshaft and passivate the system, retract the driveshaft approximately 1 cm once proximal to the lesion. Visualization under fluoroscopy of the burr retracting indicates that the tension has been relieved (Figure 3.24).

If tension or compression on the system is not relieved prior to activation, the burr will lurch forward when the device is activated. This uncontrolled forward lurch of the burr may exert significant pressure in contact with the tissue and the lesion. This may result in thermal damage, generation of larger particles, and potentially a torsional dissection.

Figure 3.25 A&B

Platforming the Burr

A) Graphic illustration of the proper method to platform the burr prior to treatment. Advance the burr proximal to the lesion site (top). Then pull or retract the driveshaft and burr assembly back slightly to relieve driveshaft compression (bottom).

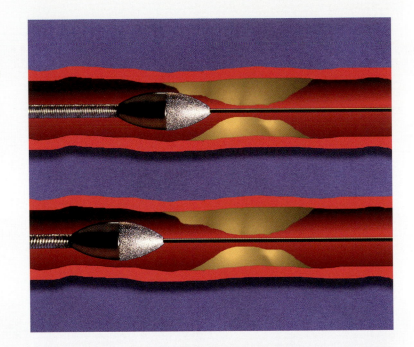

B) After the driveshaft has been decompressed, use contrast injections (top) to visualize the relative positions of the burr and lesion, and to insure that there is adequate clearance around the burr.

Once these precautions have been taken, activate the burr and begin ablation, (bottom).

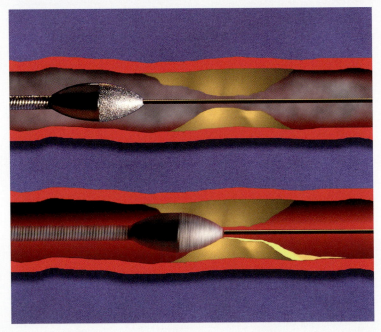

Platforming the Burr

The burr should now be positioned approximately 1 cm proximal to the lesion (Figure 3.25). This is designated as the platform segment. The burr should not be in contact with the arterial wall. This is verified by dye, which should flow unobstructed around the burr. If there is reduced flow, the burr should be repositioned more proximally to assure a free or unimpeded rotation when activated. If a free segment cannot be attained, then the burr may be too large, and exchanging to a smaller size should be considered.

Finally, set the platform speed according to burr size by adjusting the pressure on the console.

Setting Burr Speeds According to Burr Size

Larger burrs have higher surface velocities for a given rpm than smaller burrs (Figure 3.26). Therefore, when activating the device in the platform segment, the burr speed is adjusted according to

Platform Speed

The baseline speed set in the platform segment prior to advancing the burr.

Platform Speeds:
- 180,000 rpm for burrs ≤ 2.0 mm
- 160,000 rpm for burrs ≥ 2.15 mm

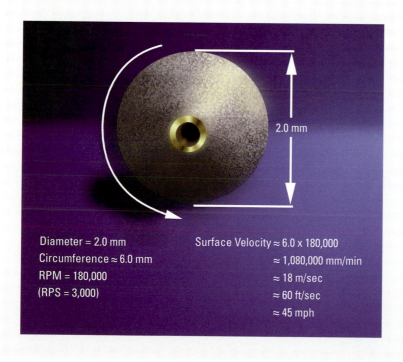

Diameter = 2.0 mm
Circumference ≈ 6.0 mm
RPM = 180,000
(RPS = 3,000)

Surface Velocity ≈ 6.0 x 180,000
≈ 1,080,000 mm/min
≈ 18 m/sec
≈ 60 ft/sec
≈ 45 mph

2.0 mm

Figure 3.26

Calculation of Surface Velocity of the Burr

Surface velocity depends on burr size and rpm. Because larger burrs have a higher surface velocity than smaller burrs at the same rpm, the platform speed for larger burrs is slightly lower. The platform speed for burrs ≤ 2.0 mm is 180,000 rpm and for burrs ≥ 2.15 mm is 160,000 rpm. Lower speeds (140,000–160,000) can be used for treatment if desired. Refer to product labeling for recommended rotational speeds.

Figure 3.27 A&B

Proper Ablation Technique

A) After platforming about 1 cm proximal to the lesion (top) the lesion is ablated. The burr engages the lesion for 2–3 seconds (middle) and then is retracted briefly for restoration of flow (lower) oscillating back and forth as it advances through the lesion. A single run is 15–30 seconds and it is not necessary to completely ablate the lesion in a single run.

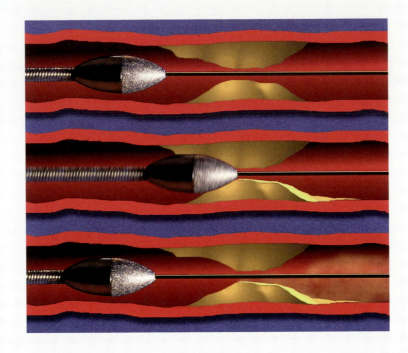

size. Platform speed for smaller burrs (≤ 2.0 mm) is 180,000 rpm and for larger burrs (≥ 2.15 mm) is 160,000 rpm. The rpm are increased or decreased by the technician at the console. Before advancing to engage the lesion, the operator should note this speed as the baseline rpm level or platform speed.

Occasionally a burr cannot reach the predesignated speed in the platform segment despite adequate air pressure to the console. One or more of the following reasons may apply: significant tortuosity in the coronary tree; multiple exchanges over the guidewire reducing the amount of lubrication; a kink in the guidewire; or a guide catheter that is not coaxial. Possible solutions include repositioning the guide catheter or exchanging the guidewire. The burr can function at lower speeds, but ablation of the plaque may take longer. Several operators are studying lower rpm treatment to determine if the decreased heat generation and platelet activation

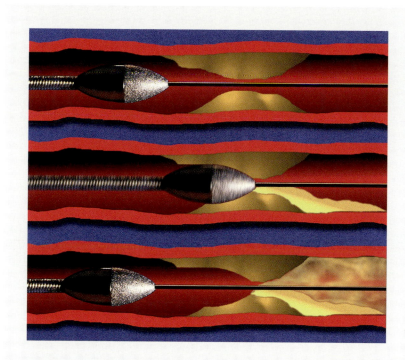

Figure 3.27 B
continued

Improper Ablation Technique

B) Continuously advancing the burr (middle image), rather than oscillating, increases the risk of excessive heat generation and of a large bolus of atherothrombotic debris (bottom image).

observed at these speeds in vitro will result in clinical benefit. Adjusting for a lower rpm is different than being unable to attain the desired speed. The latter potentially indicates a problem in the system which needs to be addressed before proceeding.

Ablation Technique

One of the major advances in procedural technique has been the refinement of lesion ablation.

After the device has been activated in the platform segment and the baseline speed has been adjusted, the burr is then gently advanced through the lesion. The movement of the burr should be dictated by the feedback of several integrating factors: the change in rpm which occurs almost simultaneously with a change in the pitch or sound of the device, the visual assessment of the movement of the burr through the diseased segment and the clinical and

Minimize Decelerations

Maintain the burr speed within 5,000 rpm of the platform speed.

hemodynamic parameters of the patient.

The ablation technique (Figure 3.27) is to slowly and gently engage the lesion with the rotating burr and slowly retract (oscillating technique). After approximately 10 seconds, a dye injection should be performed to interrogate flow and cutting orientation. The burr should be adequately retracted to permit restoration of flow down the vessel. Retracting the burr has several benefits, including:

- Restoring flow and reducing ischemia time.
- Allowing the dilution of particles by antegrade coronary blood flow, and potentially avoiding a large bolus of particles.
- Cooling of the device by withdrawing the burr into a fluid filled segment which acts as a heat-sink.
- Permitting assessment of the distal bed for slow flow or vasospasm with a simultaneous contrast injection.

RPM Surveillance

One of the most important criteria for proper ablation is careful maintenance of the speed within 5,000 rpm of the baseline or platform speed. A significant drop in speed is most likely due to aggressive advancement of the device (increased tissue pressure), results in generation of significant heat (see Chapter 1, page 16) and is a predictor of adverse events (see Chapter 2, page 30). Therefore, the operator must be extremely gentle and patient when progressing forward through the lesion. A significant drop in speed (greater than 20,000 rpm) during a slow, progressive ablation may be secondary to a guidewire with an intramural position or to an oversized burr. The burr should be retracted to assess the situation.

Vessel tortuosity may affect device speed. In certain cases, advancing the burr around a bend in a "non-diseased" segment may decrease the speed. Free flowing contrast around the burr confirms the tortuosity as the cause of the deceleration. When the rpm drop is a result of tortuosity, then a new baseline is established and staying within 5,000 rpm of that new baseline is acceptable. Any time the device is spinning unimpeded in a lumen larger than the burr size, this rpm level can be established as a new platform speed.

Visual Feedback

Ablation is a dynamic process and differs from other devices which are basically delivered to the treatment site and applied. During burr activation, intermittent visual assessment with contrast injection provides important information to the operator as the burr advances through the vessel (Figure 3.28). This critical data includes the progress of the burr through the lesion, burr interaction in segments with tortuosity and angulation, distal tapering of the vessel, presence of guidewire bias, and the relation of the burr to the size of the artery. Visual assessment can also provide an early warning mechanism for the presence of vasospasm or attenuated distal flow as the harbinger of slow flow.

Visual Assessment

Consider the burr a scalpel and the guidewire a surgeon's hand directing the cut.

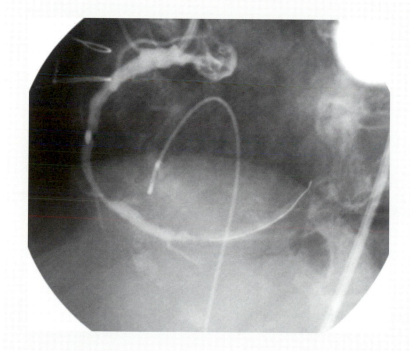

Figure 3.28

Visual Assessment

Case Information:
- Guide Catheter: 9 Fr Hockeystick
- Guidewire: Type C
- Pacemaker: Yes
- Burrs: 1.5, 2.0, 2.25 mm
- PTCA: 3.5 x 30 mm @ 1atm

After treating with a 2.0 mm burr, a 2.25 mm burr would not advance distally to the lesion without excessive decelerations due to heavy calcium and guidewire bias. Visual assessment of the burr during ablation provides information on the sizing and tracking of the burr.

Figure 3.29 A&B

Visual Assessment of Anatomical Landmarks

Case Information:
- Guide Catheter: 8 Fr JL-4
- Guidewire: Type C
- Pacemaker: No
- Burrs: 1.75, 2.15 mm
- PTCA: 3.0 x 30 mm perfusion

A) These restenotic lesions (arrows) in the LAD of a 79 year-old male were treated with a 1.75 mm burr followed by a 2.15 mm burr. The 1.75 mm burr was selected as the initial burr because the lesions were restenotic. In de novo lesions a 1.5 mm burr would have been chosen as the initial burr.

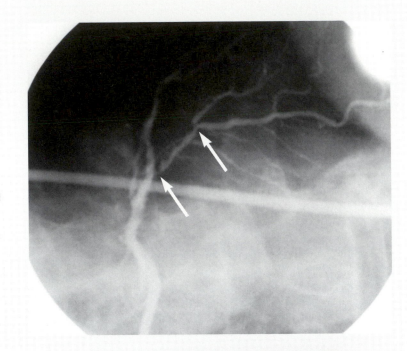

B) The 2.15 mm burr was mistakenly advanced beyond the distal lesion site into the small tapering vessel resulting in perforation. The perforation (arrow) was treated with a 3.0 mm perfusion balloon. Visual contrast assessment can provide identification for anatomical landmarks for the position of the burr and prevent such complications.

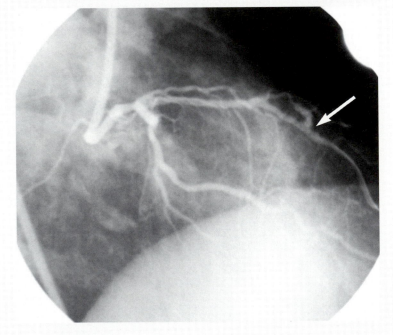

The following are helpful applications for visual assessment during an ablation sequence:

- Burr deceleration: visualization of the burr location can explain whether the drop in speed is due to overaggressive advancement into the lesion or vessel tortuosity. In the case of vessel tortuosity, contrast will flow unimpeded around the burr.
- Guidewire bias: visualization of the burr as it advances may demonstrate the orientation of the burr preferentially to one surface. This orientation may affect the result achieved with the burr and influence subsequent sizing.
- Segmental ablation: long and heavily calcified lesions do not have to be completely treated in one run sequence. Contrast injections can help monitor progress through the lesion, and provide identification as to anatomical landmarks for subsequent ablations (Figure 3.29).
- Obstructive burr: when ablating a lesion, the flow should not be totally obstructed for more than a few seconds. If there is no antegrade flow around the burr, during a contrast injection, retract the device until the contrast completely clears the vessel.

Ablation Time

One controversial aspect of rotational atherectomy is the time of ablation. The ablation time should allow for adequate engagement of the lesion for removal of plaque, balanced with the ability of the distal bed to clear the particles (Figure 3.30).

Presently, ablation time intervals of 15–30 seconds are recommended. Often several runs are required to completely cross a lesion. This is referred to as segmental ablation.

Interval Between Ablation Runs

Allowing time to elapse between ablation runs is important to provide time for particle clearance. In addition, the operator can identify immediately any negative sequelae such as slow flow or vasospasm that may have occurred during the treatment. Between

Segmental Ablation

Uses several runs lasting between 15–30 seconds to complete treatment of a lesion.

Figure 3.30 A&B

Ablation Time

Case Information:
- Guide Catheter: 9 Fr JL-4
- Guidewire: Type C
- Pacemaker: No
- Burrs: 1.75, 2.15 mm
- PTCA: 3.5 x 30 mm
  @ 1.5 atm

A) This 55 year-old man with stable angina had a mid 90% 15 mm LAD lesion (arrow). It was dilated to 18 atm without significant reduction in stenosis severity. Since there was no angiographic evidence of intimal disruption, a decision was made to treat with rotational atherectomy.

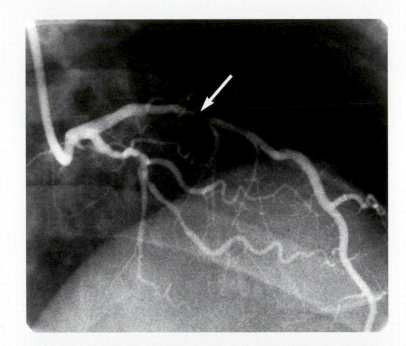

B) The vessel was treated with 1.75 and 2.15 mm burrs. Due to the severe lesion calcification, more than 5 minutes of ablation time was required to cross the lesion. Post-atherectomy the lesion was dilated with a 3.5 mm balloon at 1.5 atm to achieve the result shown.

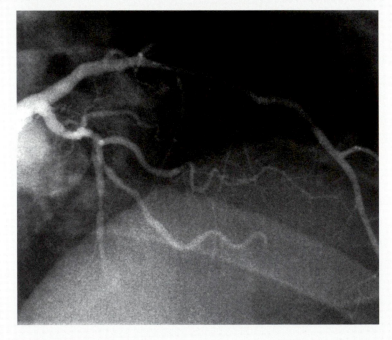

runs the burr should be retracted sufficiently for ample antegrade coronary flow. In the vast majority of cases, the time between treatments is brief (30–60 seconds), but should be modified based on hemodynamics, ECG changes and chest discomfort. The advantages of patience during the procedure cannot be overstated. This approach is particularly important in incremental, step-burr procedures. If the patient has significant ECG changes, or severe chest pain, a larger device should not be introduced until these parameters are normalized. This process may take 5–20 minutes. Between ablation runs vasodilators, manual blood perfusion, or other corrective measures such as low-pressure PTCA can be used as required (see Chapter 7, pages 247–248). In the majority of cases, chest pain and ECG changes resolve spontaneously.

Polishing Run
The final ablation run called the "polishing run" should be associated with no drop in rpm and no perception of mechanical resistance as the burr crosses the treated segment.

Primary Therapy vs. Lesion Modification
Primary therapy is defined as achieving maximal safe debulking with the device followed by no further adjunctive therapy (rare) or the use of an oversized balloon at low pressures (greater by 0.5 mm than would be used therapeutically at less than or equal to one atmosphere). The balloon in these cases is predominantly indicated to relieve vasospasm, or improve the angiographic hazy appearance that is often seen immediately after rotational atherectomy. The burr-to-artery ratio in these cases is in the range of 0.70–0.85. The ability to achieve a primary therapy strategy is often limited by lesion characteristics, proximal tortuosity (making it difficult to safely advance larger burrs to the lesion), limited distal runoff, or clinical parameters such as poor left ventricular function. Those lesion morphologies that are applicable to this approach are those without severe angulation, i.e. straight segments, or those

with favorable guidewire characteristics where larger burrs can be applied. Intraprocedural factors may alter the strategy such as significant unremitting chest pain, or ECG changes after the initial burr. Larger burrs should not be used in a patient demonstrating these unstable clinical parameters.

Lesion modification is defined as the use of rotational atherectomy to improve the lesion and luminal characteristics in order to apply adjunctive technologies including PTCA, directional atherectomy (DCA) and stents. Several reports have supported the ability of the Rotablator to change the vessel compliance and therefore work synergistically with other devices.[57,58,66] This strategy can be planned for cases where the vessel, lesion or left ventricular function are suboptimal for the deployment of larger burrs. Lesion modification can also be applied with the goal of achieving minimal residual stenosis. The burr-to-artery ratio in these cases can vary based on the adjunctive therapy (PTCA, directional atherectomy, or stenting) applied, but should be significant enough that the advantages of the device synergy are realized. For example, in the case of rotastent, the Rotablator can potentially increase vessel and lesion compliance and symmetry for improved delivery, deployment and concentric apposition of stents. What burr-to-artery ratio is required to reap the benefits from rotational atherectomy in not precisely known, but debulking of greater than a 0.6 burr-to-artery ratio is recommended.

Primary Therapy vs. Lesion Modification Case Studies
These case studies provide insight into the types of anatomy that favor either primary therapy or lesion modification. At present the decision is dictated solely by acute outcome. Ongoing studies that focus on long-term outcome may define optimal debulking and adjunctive therapy strategies. (Text resumes on page 104.)

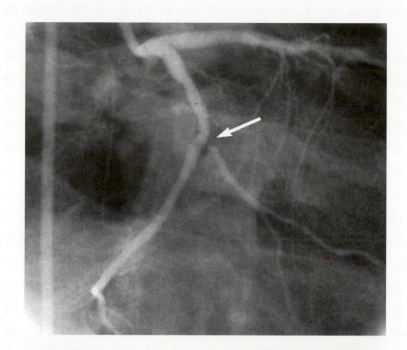

Figure 3.31 A&B

Primary Therapy

Case Information:
- Guide Catheter: 8 Fr JL-4
- Guidewire: Type C
- Pacemaker: No
- Burrs: 1.5, 2.0 mm
- PTCA: No

A) This 55 year-old male, with two prior angioplasties of the proximal circumflex returned with a 95% stenosis of the first obtuse marginal branch (arrow). An ACS HI-Torque Floppy guidewire was used to cross the lesion followed by exchange for the Type C guidewire. The lesion was treated using 1.5 and 2.0 mm burrs.

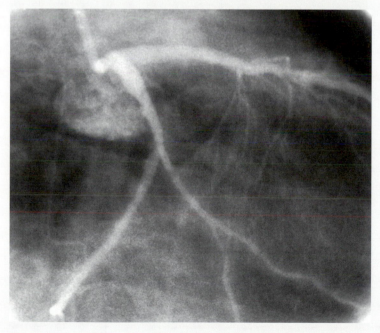

B) Following atherectomy there was less than 10% residual stenosis. Adjunctive PTCA was not necessary.

Figure 3.32 A&B

Therapy After Failed PTCA

Case Information:
- Guide Catheter: 8 Fr JL-4
- Guidewire: Type C
- Pacemaker: No
- Burrs: 1.5, 2.0 mm
- PTCA: 2.5 @ 1 atm

A) The mid circumflex lesion (arrow) in this 78 year-old was attempted with a 2.5 mm balloon at 8 atm without any change in stenosis severity.

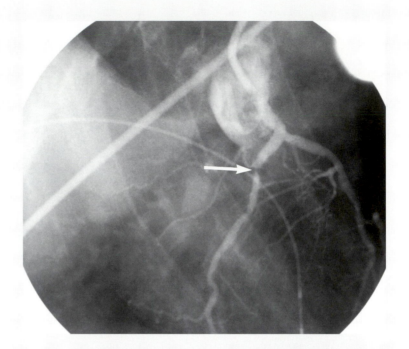

B) Subsequent treatment with the Rotablator system using 1.5 and 2.0 mm burrs followed by a 2.5 mm balloon at 1 atm yielded an excellent result.

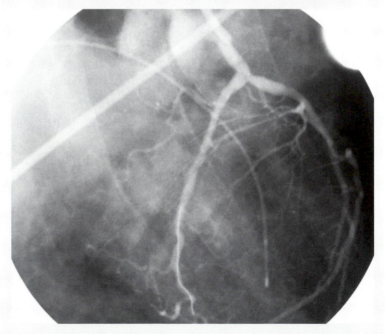

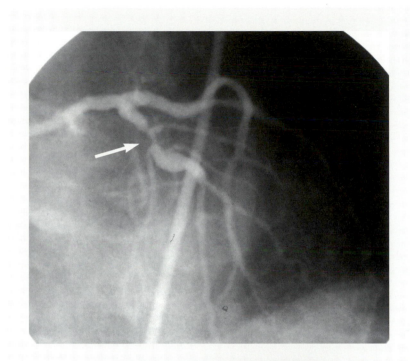

Figure 3.33 A&B

**Lesion Modification
with Stenting**

Case Information:
- Guide Catheter: 9 Fr JL-4
- Guidewire: Type C, Extra
  Support
- Pacemaker: No
- Burrs: 1.5, 2.0 mm
- Stent: PS 1530
- PTCA 3.5 mm (post-stent)

A) This 68 year-old male
presented with progressive
angina and a heavily calcified
mid-LAD lesion followed by an
ectatic area (arrow). The lesion
was treated with 1.5 mm and
2.0 mm burrs. The guidewire
was vectored superiorly
precluding the use of larger
burrs.

B) Post-atherectomy a
PS 1530 stent was implanted
(arrow) and dilated to 18 atm
with a 3.5 mm balloon.

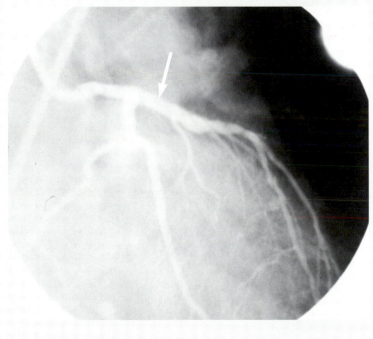

Figure 3.34 A-D

Lesion Modification with DCA

Case Information:
- Guide Catheter: 9 Fr JR-4
- Guidewire: Type C
- Pacemaker: Yes
- Burrs: 1.5, 2.0 mm
- DCA: Proximal-RCA
- PTCA: 3.5 x 20 mm
  @ 2 atm

A) This 72 year-old man had severe stenoses in the proximal and mid-RCA which was heavily calcified and tortuous.

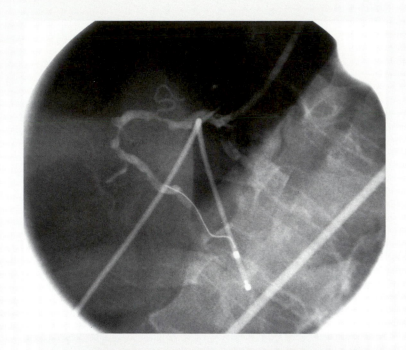

B) Rotational atherectomy was performed using 1.5 and 2.0 mm burrs to remove superficial calcium.

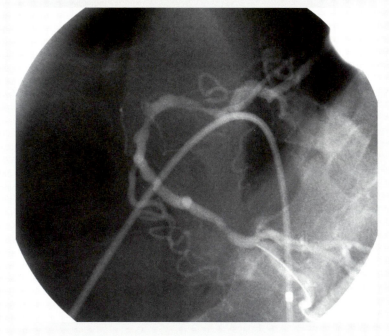

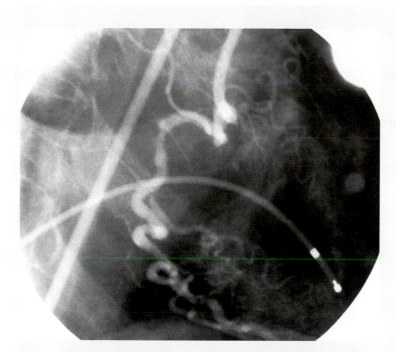

Figure 3.34 C&D
continued

C) After rotational atherectomy the proximal lesion was treated with directional coronary atherectomy (DCA).

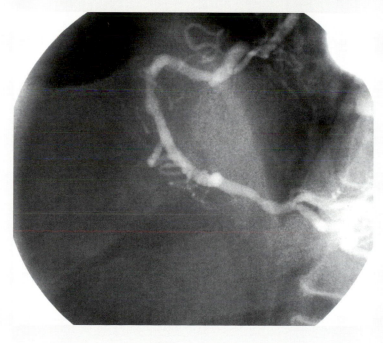

D) Adjunctive PTCA was performed with a 3.5 mm balloon.

Adjunctive PTCA Post High-Speed Rotational Atherectomy

One suggested method of adjunctive PTCA in patients treated with primary therapy, consists of using a balloon oversized by 0.5 mm greater than the size ordinarily used for primary therapeutic PTCA at low-pressure inflations (≤ 1 atm). This technique for adjunctive balloon angioplasty is recommended to:

- Reduce the possibility of inducing intimal tears or deep medial wall injury.
- Relieve vasospasm.
- "Tack down" any "intimal disruptions".

The rationale for this strategy is derived from Lame's equation which states that the wall tension at a given pressure is increased as a multiple of the lumen size and is inversely proportional to the wall thickness. Therefore, the wall tension following rotational atherectomy, at any given pressure, is significantly increased due to plaque removal producing a larger lumen and decreasing the wall thickness (Figure 3.35).

In most cases, low-pressure inflations, appear to increase luminal dimensions, reduce post-ablation haziness and can mechanically "break" vasospasm. When significantly undersized burrs are used (e.g. with severe vessel angles) higher pressures for a sufficient increase in luminal dimensions are needed (lesion modification strategy). If the angiographic result is unsatisfactory after use of a low-pressure inflation, it is acceptable to proceed with a larger burr as described below. In cases of lesion modification conventional pressures are used with appropriately sized balloons.

Rotational Atherectomy following Primary PTCA

Rotational atherectomy following attempted PTCA is an acceptable method of treatment. This strategy has been limited to those lesions with an inadequate result and no angiographic evidence of dissection post-balloon inflation. One strategy to avoid dissections

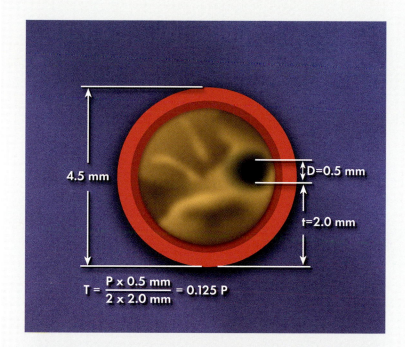

4.5 mm

↕ D=0.5 mm

t=2.0 mm

$$T = \frac{P \times 0.5 \text{ mm}}{2 \times 2.0 \text{ mm}} = 0.125 \text{ P}$$

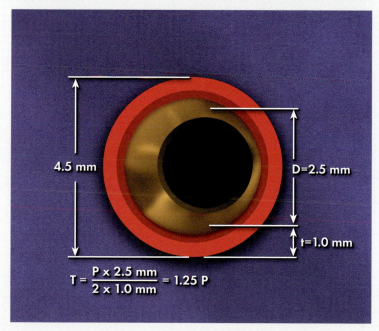

4.5 mm

D=2.5 mm

t=1.0 mm

$$T = \frac{P \times 2.5 \text{ mm}}{2 \times 1.0 \text{ mm}} = 1.25 \text{ P}$$

Figure 3.35 A&B

Lame's Equation

Originally developed to determine the pressure of steam in pipes, Lame's equation describes tension in a pressurized cylinder as being proportional to the thickness of the cylinder wall. This equation is used to determine arterial wall tension.

A) The untreated vessel has a lumen of 0.5 mm in an artery that originally had an inner diameter of 3.0 mm and outer diameter of 4.5 mm. Using Lame's equation (where "P" is pressure and "T" is tension), the tension on the wall will be 0.125 times the lumen pressure.

B) After treatment with rotational atherectomy, the lumen has been enlarged, and conversely, the vessel thickness has been reduced. By factoring in the new dimensions, the tension in the treated vessel wall is calculated at 1.25 P. Pressures applied within each vessel (via PTCA for example) will be 10 times higher in the treated vessel as compared to the untreated vessel.

is to limit pressures to 6 atms (usually 4 atms). If a waist is still present in the balloon, implying a noncompliant lesion, remove the balloon and evaluate the lesion angiographically. If no dissection is evident, proceed with rotational atherectomy. After debulking, even at low burr-to-artery ratios (below 0.6) the balloon, when reinserted, will often achieve nominal size at 2–6 atm of pressure. If not, a larger burr can be placed and the sequence repeated (see Figures 3.37, 3.38 and 3.39). This is an excellent way to assess lesion compliance ("poor man's IVUS") and may, for example, potentially predict the ability of a stent to be adequately deployed.

Interpolated Angioplasty

Interpolated angioplasty is a recent advancement aimed at optimizing rotational atherectomy results. It refers to the ability to use PTCA as an intermediate step between deciding on the use of incremental burrs. After the initial burr, PTCA at low to moderate pressures (2–6 atms) can provide information about lesion compliance. It can also be a treatment for vasospasm or slow flow. After the PTCA, if larger burr sizes are indicated, they may be used assuming no evidence of dissection and resumption of TIMI III flow (see Figure 3.40).

PTCA with Rotational Atherectomy Case Studies

Device synergy is a methodology to achieve a favorable outcome. The mechanism of debulking and arterial expansion with PTCA and stents frequently can be merged to maximize the potential of these devices. The following case studies demonstrate the synergistic use of these devices to achieve successful outcomes. (Text resumes on page 117.)

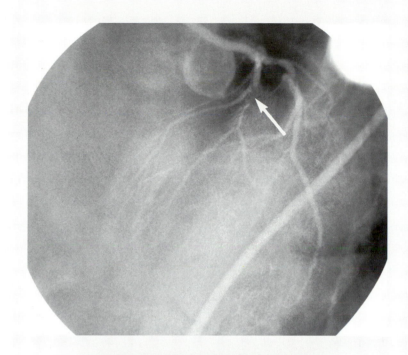

Figure 3.36 A&B

**Rotational Atherectomy
with Adjunctive PTCA**

Case Information:
- Guide Catheter: 9 Fr FL-4
- Guidewire: Type C
- Pacemaker: No
- Burrs: 1.25, 1.5 mm
- PTCA: 2.5 x 20 mm
  @ 1 atm

A) This 58 year-old female had undergone triple vessel bypass surgery to the RCA, LAD and circumflex arteries with only the RCA remaining patent. Several guidewires were used before the subtotal occlusion in the LAD (arrow) was crossed with a Silk guidewire. The distal tip of the guidewire was placed in the diagonal artery.

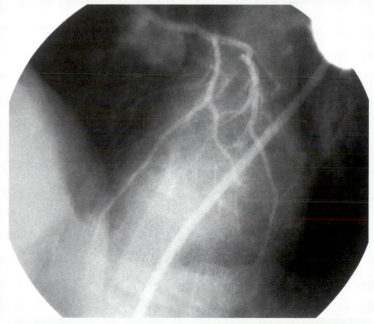

B) After exchange for the Type C wire, the proximal LAD and the diagonal were treated with 1.25 and 1.5 mm burrs. With some difficulty the guidewire was redirected into the distal LAD and the mid-LAD was treated with 1.25 and 1.5 mm burrs.

Adjunctive PTCA was performed with a 2.5 mm balloon advanced into the distal LAD and inflated to 1 atm beginning in the distal LAD area and continuing proximally yielding an excellent result.

Figure 3.37 A-D

Rotational Atherectomy After Failed PTCA

Case Information:
- Guide Catheter: 8 Fr JL-4
- Guidewire: Type C
- Pacemaker: No
- Burrs: 1.75
- PTCA: 2.5 mm @ 2 atm

A) PTCA was the intended treatment for this stenosis in the mid LAD (arrow).

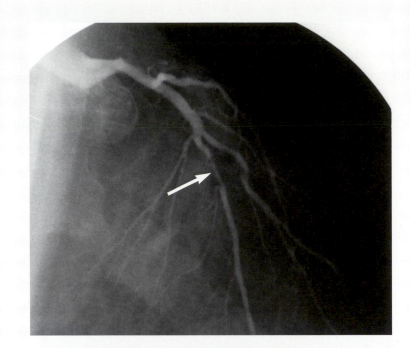

B) A 2.5 x 2.0 mm balloon at 6 atm did not fully inflate (arrow) indicating probable occult calcification. Since there was no apparent dissection, the Choice™ guidewire was exchanged for a Type C guidewire.

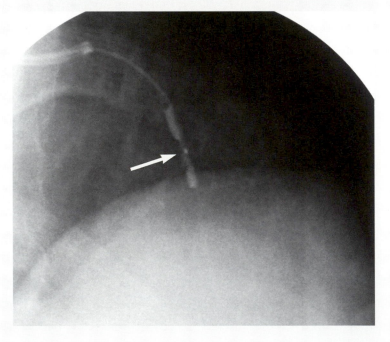

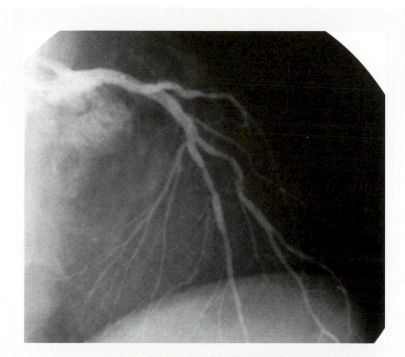

Figure 3.37 C&D
continued

C) A 1.75 mm burr was used to debulk the lesion and to increase vessel compliance. A 1.75 mm burr was selected since the lumen had been expanded by PTCA. Had the case been planned for rotational atherectomy the burr selection would have been 1.5 mm followed by a 2.0 mm burr.

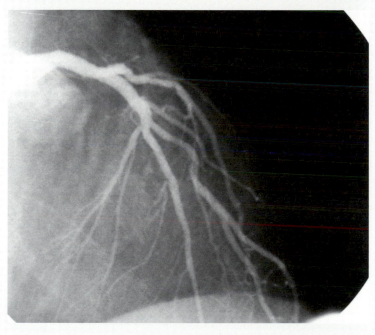

D) Following debulking the 2.5 x 20 mm balloon was fully expanded at 2 atm with an excellent final result.

Figure 3.38 A-D

**Rotational Atherectomy
After Failed PTCA**

Case Information:
- Guide Catheter: 8 Fr JR-4
- Guidewire: RotaWire
  Floppy
- Pacemaker: Yes
- Burrs: 1.5, 1.75 mm
- PTCA: 3.0 x 30 mm
  @ 6 atm and 2 atm

A) Treatment of the distal
RCA (arrow) in a 79 year-old
man was planned for PTCA.

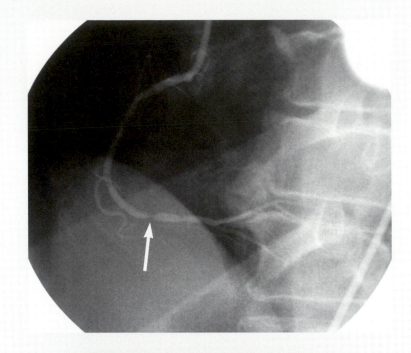

B) PTCA of the vessel at 6
atm demonstrated a balloon
waist (arrow). The balloon and
guidewire were exchanged
and the lesion was treated
with 1.5 and 1.75 mm burrs.

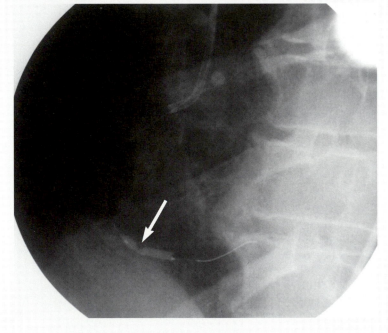

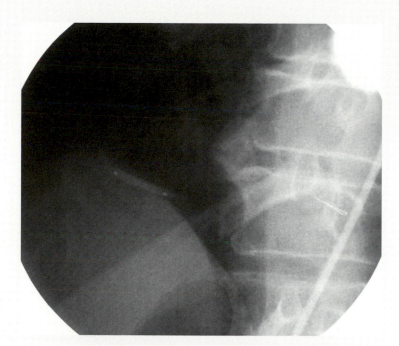

Figure 3.38 C&D
continued

C) Post-atherectomy the balloon was fully expanded at 2 atm.

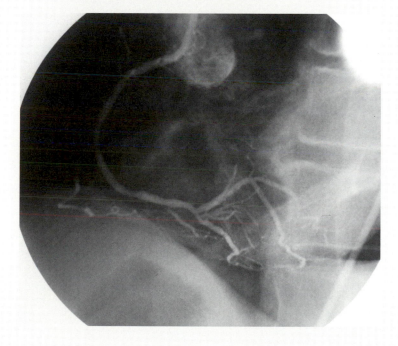

D) Final residual stenosis was < 20%.

Figure 3.39 A-D

**Rotational Atherectomy
After Failed PTCA**

Case Information:
- Guide Catheter: 8 Fr
  Voda 3.5
- Guidewire: Choice™,
  RotaWire Floppy
- Pacemaker: No
- Burrs: 1.5 mm
- PTCA: 2.5 x 20 mm
  @ 4 atm.

A) This 77 year-old male presented with multivessel disease of the circumflex and LAD and unstable angina. The angiogram demonstrates haziness and beading at the lesion site (arrow). Because of the clinical presentation, PTCA was selected as the initial treatment.

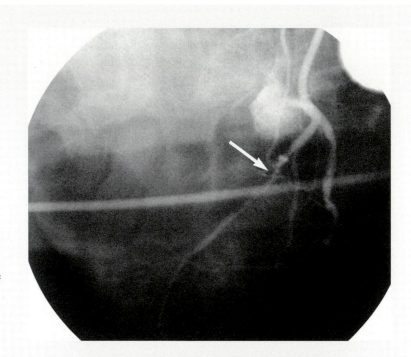

B) Inflation of the balloon to 6 atm revealed a waist (arrow) in the balloon where the lesion did not yield. In the absence of visible dissection, rotational atherectomy was used.

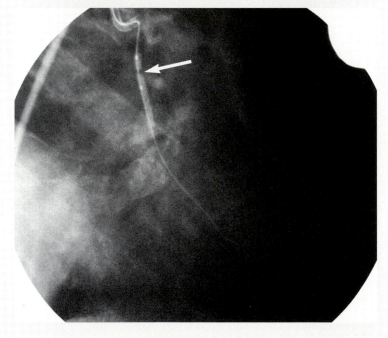

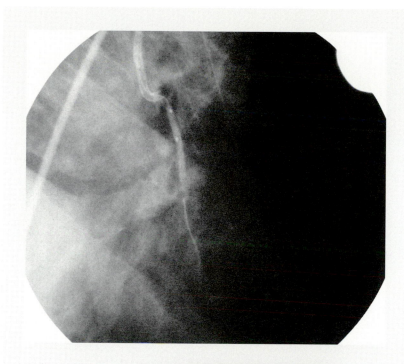

Figure 3.39 C&D
continued

C) After treatment with a 1.5 mm burr, the balloon was fully expanded at 4 atm.

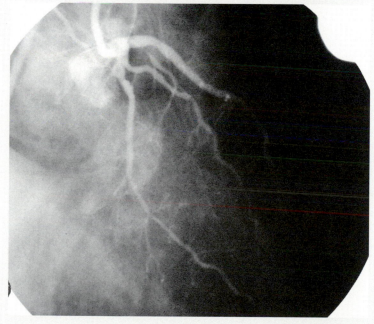

D) Post-treatment residual stenosis was < 10% and an excellent result achieved. Six weeks post-procedure the LAD was treated. The circumflex was widely patent.

Figure 3.40 A-F

Interpolated Angioplasty

Case Information:
- Guide Catheter: 8 Fr JL-4
- Guidewire: RotaWire Floppy
- Pacemaker: No
- Burrs: 1.25, 1.5, 1.75 mm
- PTCA: 2.0 x 20 mm @ 2 atm; 2.5 x 30 mm @ 4 atm

A) This 55 year-old man was admitted with unstable angina and a complex 99% stenosis of the proximal LAD.

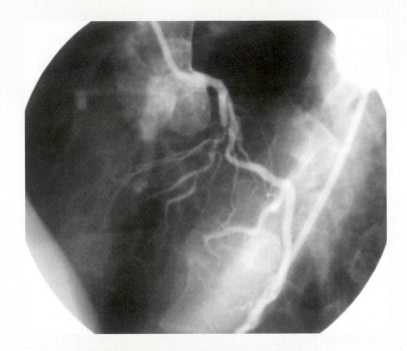

B) After crossing the lesion with the RotaWire Floppy a 1.25 mm burr was used to treat the lesion.

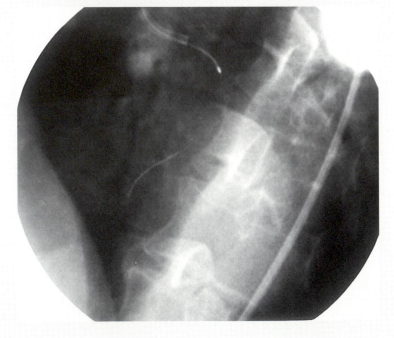

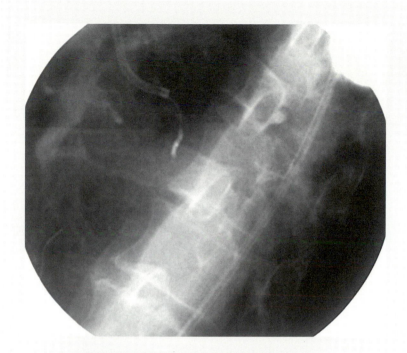

Figure 3.40 C&D
continued

C) After the 1.25 mm burr, vasospasm occurred resulting in total occlusion of the LAD which was treated with a 2.0 x 20 mm balloon at 2 atm to mechanically relieve the spasm.

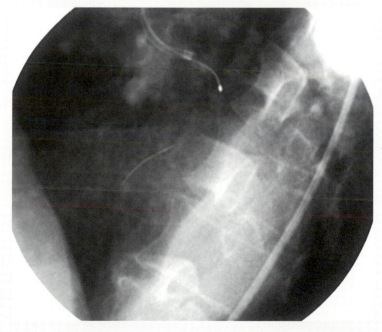

D) A 1.5 mm burr was advanced through the lesion and it was again followed by total occlusion which was treated with a 2.0 mm balloon followed by a 2.5 x 30 mm balloon at 4 atm with restoration of flow.

Figure 3.40 E&F
continued

E) After restoration of flow, a significant stenosis in the proximal vessel was still present. This was treated with a 1.75 mm burr followed by balloon inflation to 6 atm with a 2.5 mm balloon.

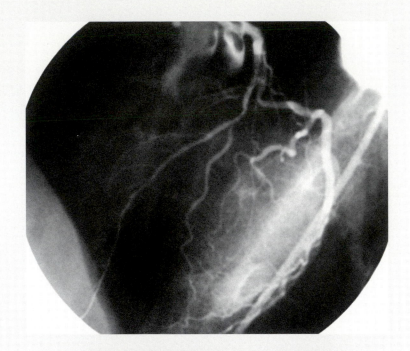

F) Because of the question of thrombus formation (haziness at the site) (arrow), the patient was placed on the platelet inhibitor ReoPro and remained clinically stable.

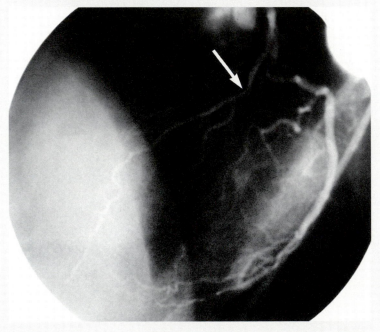

Post-Procedure Management

In preparation for transfer to a monitored setting, the intravascular sheaths are sutured in place, topical or intravenous nitroglycerin is continued, and fluids (normal saline) are infused to maintain adequate hydration. The pacemaker is removed unless bradyarrythmias persist after therapy (this occurrence is rare).

Occasionally the patient may experience persistent chest pain and electrocardiographic abnormalities including ST elevation or depression post-procedure. This can occur despite a coronary angiogram that demonstrates an excellent result with TIMI-3 flow and patency of all the arterial branches. Typically, the pain diminishes and is relieved with normalization of the ST-T wave segments within 20 minutes. Obtaining a baseline for the intensity of pain is important in order to determine if a patient's symptoms have deteriorated.

Patients should be monitored in a telemetry setting overnight. In addition to intravenous nitroglycerin and fluids, aspirin and calcium channel blockers are administered. Intravascular sheaths are maintained overnight but, based on the angiographic result, this decision can be left to operator discretion.

The issue of anticoagulation is controversial. In uncomplicated cases, continuation of heparin is often unnecessary. Patients with excessively long lesions or total occlusions, and patients with evidence of dissection or thrombus, may benefit from the use of prolonged anticoagulation.

Treatment by Vessel

Chapter 4

The content and format in this section is organized as a reference to aid the interventional cardiologist in the catheterization laboratory to unique aspects of rotational atherectomy. Specific topics covered include clinical issues, equipment recommendations, burr selection, technique and implementation of adjunctive devices. The discussion in this chapter focuses on treatment of lesions by vessel. In subsequent chapters lesion characteristics and lesion locations are covered.

Left Anterior Descending Artery

The left anterior descending artery was the most frequently treated vessel from the multicenter registry.[67] Special considerations when treating the left anterior descending include the occasional need to platform in the left main artery and the need to assess disease and flow in the diagonals prior to the intervention. The RAO with significant cranial orientation is an exceptional view to demonstrate the relationships between the left main, the proximal or ostial LAD and the trajectory of the burr. Frequent contrast injections can aid in the assessment of the presence or absence of vasospasm in the branching diagonals.

Guide Catheter
- Select a guide catheter (with sideholes) that is large enough to accommodate the largest anticipated burr.
- Attempt to avoid shapes that are directed to the roof of the left

main since this may hinder burr advancement.

- Coaxial placement is more important than firm intubation.

Guidewire

- The Type C or RotaWire Extra Support guidewires are generally used, because they provide greater vessel contact with eccentric lesions in straight segments.
- In proximal lesions, assess guidewire bias due to the trajectory from the guide catheter.
- In treating proximal lesions with distal tortuosity, the RotaWire Floppy guidewire adds advantages.

Pacemaker

- A temporary pacemaker is recommended when treating ostial LAD lesions with burrs 2.25 mm and greater.

Burr Selection

- A stepped-burr approach is recommended.
- Due to the often large size of the vessel adjunctive therapy may be required to minimize residual stenosis.

Ablation Technique

- Use gentle advancement avoiding decelerations greater than 5,000 rpm and keep ablation times to 15–30 sec./run.
- In proximal lesions it may be necessary to platform in the left main coronary artery. No adverse sequelae have been noted.
- The LAD often tapers rapidly. Contrast injections help to assess the transition to smaller segments. (Figure 3.20, page 78).

Strategy

- Proximal segments are commonly treated with a rotastent technique.
- Assessment of the presence or absence of disease in the diagonals is important since vasospasm post-rotational atherectomy may direct the operator into mechanical intervention when only vasodilators are required.
- In the presence of an occluded RCA , treating LAD lesions with large territories are considered higher risk.[60]

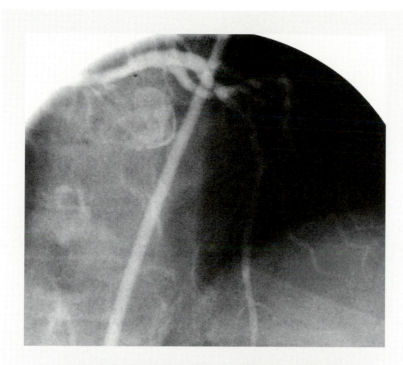

Figure 4.1 A&B

LAD Lesion Involving a Nondiseased Sidebranch

Case Information:
- Guide Catheter: 9 Fr JL-4
- Guidewire: Type C
- Pacemaker: No
- Burrs: 1.75 mm
- PTCA: 3.5 x 20 mm @1.5 atm

A) Treatment of these complex lesions in the proximal and mid portions of the LAD artery was completed with a 1.75 mm burr followed by an oversized balloon at low pressure.

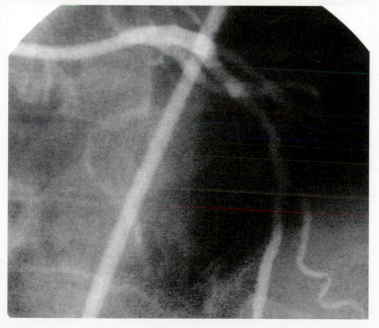

B) Final angiography revealed less than 10% residual stenosis. No vasospasm or plaque shifting was noted in the small diagonal branch.

Left Circumflex Artery

The circumflex artery may offer unique challenges especially in the management of ostial disease. The LAO caudal is often an excellent angiographic view to demonstrate the relationship of the guide catheter, guidewire and lesion for ostial circumflex lesions. In addition, due to the frequent tortuosity of the obtuse marginal branches, the guidewire will often not lie centrally.

Guide Catheter
- Select a guide catheter (with sideholes) that is large enough to accommodate the largest anticipated burr.
- An Amplatz guide catheter provides a coaxial advantage especially in the context of a short left main coronary artery for burr advancement and a centrally-oriented guidewire.

Guidewire
- Guidewire tethering can occur in tortuous obtuse marginals when advancing a nonactivated burr. Assessing placement with contrast injections and relieving the tension in the guidewire after burr advancement is recommended.

Burr Selection
- A stepped-burr approach is recommended.
- Tortuous obtuse marginals with lesions on bends may limit the use of large burrs due to significant guidewire bias. Assessing luminal gains after each burr size is important.

Pacemaker
- A temporary pacemaker is recommended in cases with left dominant circulation or when treating the circumflex artery in the presence of a right coronary occlusion.

Ablation Technique
- It may be necessary to use activated advancement techniques to advance the burr in tortuous obtuse marginal branches.
- Use gentle advancement avoiding decelerations greater than 5,000 rpm and keep ablation times to 15–30 sec./run.
- Ostial circumflex lesions often veer off at severe angles from the

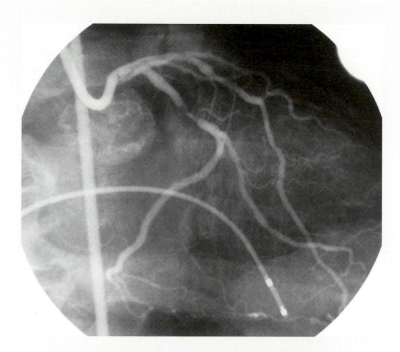

Figure 4.2 A&B

Mid-Circumflex Lesion

Case Information:
- Guide Catheter: 10 Fr JCL
- Guidewire: Type C
- Pacemaker: Yes
- Burrs: 1.75, 2.25 mm
- PTCA: No

A) This 62 year-old man presented with increasing exertional angina and was found to have a 95% stenosis of the mid circumflex artery. The lesion was treated with 1.75 and 2.25 mm burrs.

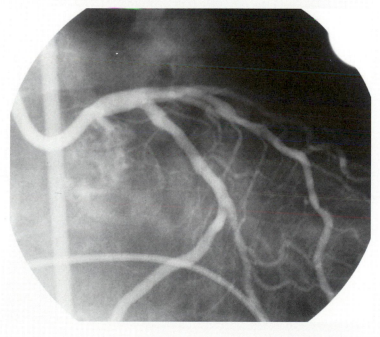

B) Following atherectomy, with the results shown, no further treatment was applied.

Figure 4.3 A-C

Calcified Circumflex Lesion

Case Information:
- Guide Catheter: 8 Fr JL-4
- Guidewire: Type C
- Pacemaker: Yes
- Burrs: 1.5, 2.0 mm
- PTCA: 3.5 x 20 mm
- Stent: PS1535

A) This 44 year-old diabetic underwent bypass surgery 12 years prior and now presented with recurrent angina. While the distal branches of the LAD and RCA served by grafts are patent, the proximal and mid-segments are diffusely diseased. The ungrafted circumflex had heavily calcified lesions (arrows).

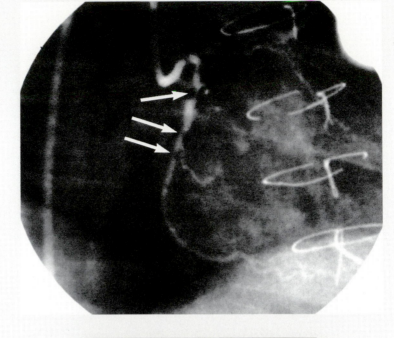

B) The lesions were treated with rotational atherectomy using 1.5 and 2.0 mm burrs to increase vessel compliance and ease deployment of the stent to the lesion site. The proximal site had moderate vasospasm after treatment.

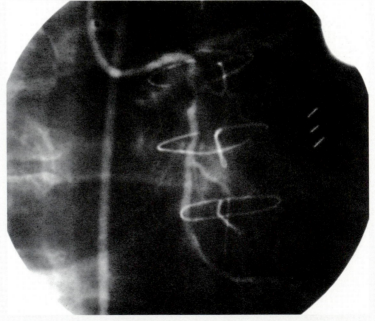

left main and a conservative approach, maintaining a low burr-to-artery ratio of 0.5–0.6 is often prudent (see Figure 4.3). Telescoping the guide catheter (often Amplatz, Voda or short-tip Judkins curves) for coaxial orientation is beneficial.

- Shortened ablation times should be performed with the onset of pacing if associated with lower diastolic blood pressure.

Strategy

- Lesion modification is preferred in severely angulated lesions due to limited burr-to-artery ratios that may be safely achieved.
- Ostial circumflex disease requires an experienced operator to interpret the appropriate guide catheter, the lie of the guidewire, the trajectory of ablation and the gains achieved after each burr.
- Circumflex arteries that originate at right angles from the left main may limit burr sizes to treat more distal disease due to guidewire bias as the burr enters the circumflex.

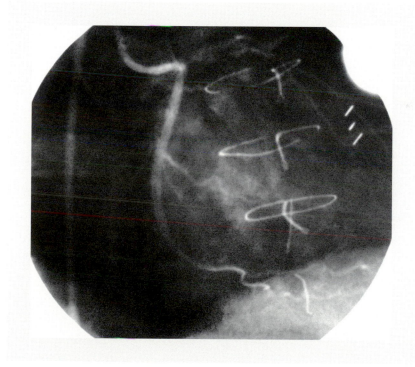

Figure 4.3 C
continued

C) The stent easily tracked around the heavily calcified circumflex and was deployed at 7 atm followed by high-pressure post-dilation.

Right Coronary Artery

The issues that are unique to the right coronary artery are the treatment of aorto-ostial disease and the frequently seen bradycardia and atrioventricular block when treating these vessels. Ellis et al.[35] demonstrated a higher incidence of slow flow in this vessel as well. This may be due to the lower coronary flow rates compared to the left circulation or to the lower diastolic pressures that are often seen with pacing.

Guide Catheter

- Select a guide catheter (with sideholes) that is large enough to accommodate the largest anticipated burr.
- Judkins and hockey-stick guides are most frequently used.
- In aorto-ostial disease (not an FDA approved indication) when it may be necessary to rotate the device in the guide catheter, selecting an "oversized" guide catheter may be beneficial.

Guidewire

- In distal lesions when support is required to advance the burr around the inferior wall of the heart, the Type C (or RotaWire Extra Support) guidewire may be superior as opposed to the RotaWire Floppy guidewire (see Figure 3.23, page 85).

Burr Selection

- A stepped-burr approach is recommended.
- Assess both the RAO and LAO views. The RAO view will often unmask significant tortuosity that may limit final burr size (see Figure 3.12, page 59).

Pacemaker

- Pacing is frequently required. In the event the pacemaker does not capture, instructing the patient to cough will often return normal sinus rhythm.

Ablation Technique

- Use gentle advancement avoiding decelerations greater than 5,000 rpm and keep ablation times to 15–30 sec./run.
- Stop ablation when the pacemaker activates and wait until

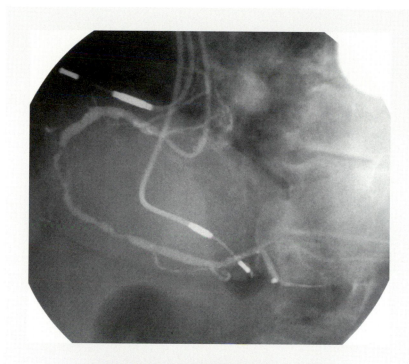

Figure 4.4 A&B
Diffusely Diseased RCA

Case Information:
- Guide Catheter: 8 Fr Amplatz
- Guidewire: Type C
- Pacemaker: Permanent
- Burrs: 1.5, 1.75 mm
- PTCA: 3.5 x 40 mm

A) Treatment of this diffusely diseased RCA in an elderly woman who was not a candidate for bypass surgery was accomplished using 1.5 and 1.75 mm burrs. Segmental ablation was performed. Three separate runs per burr were required to treat the entire lesion.

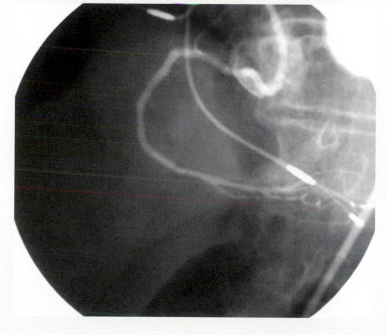

B) Adjunctive PTCA was performed with a 3.5 x 40 mm balloon at 5 atm.

Figure 4.5 A-C

Dominant RCA

Case Information:
- Guide Catheter: 8 Fr JR-4
- Guidewire: Type C
- Pacemaker: Yes
- Burrs: 1.5, 2.0 mm
- PTCA: 3.5 x 30 mm
  @ 6 atm

A) This 80 year-old man had diffuse disease and severe calcification of the dominant RCA. The platinum tip of the guidewire (arrow) was placed just distal to the angulation to avoid tethering and provide optimal freedom for the burr to become centralized.

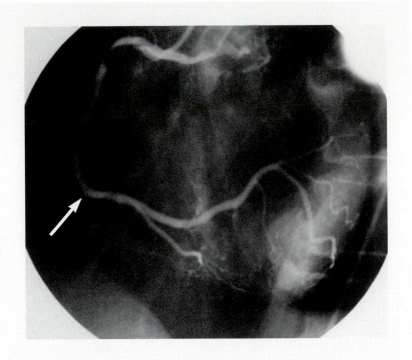

baseline rhythm returns to resume ablation.
- With the onset of pacing, shortened ablation times should be used especially if pacing is associated with lower diastolic blood pressure.

Strategy
- Vasospasm or slow flow in right ventricular branches typically are not hemodynamically problematic, but can cause significant chest discomfort, and usually improve with vasodilators and time.
- Since slow flow may be more frequent in the RCA[35], shorter runs (15 seconds) and longer intervals between runs may be indicated.
- In aorto-ostial disease with poor coaxial guide catheter placement, lesion modification with stenting has been used as a strategy. (Treatment of aorto-ostial lesions is not an FDA approved indication.)

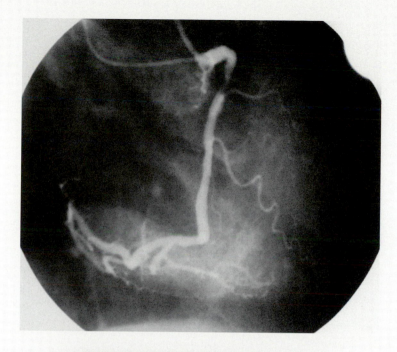

Figure 4.5 B&C
continued

B) The proximal RCA was heavily calcified and was treated with 1.5 and 2.0 mm burrs. Short ablation runs (15 sec.) were used to prevent bradycardia.

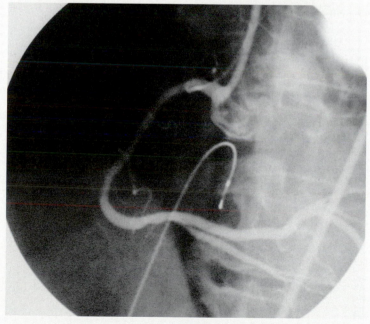

C) Post-atherectomy the vessel was treated with a 3.5 x 30 mm balloon at 1 atm and then at 6 atm. TIMI III flow was maintained throughout the procedure.

Protected Left Main Coronary Artery

Due to the fibrocalcific nature of protected left main arteries, rotational atherectomy is frequently used in this lesion type.[67] The challenging feature of treating this lesion subset includes obtaining a coaxial guide catheter position. Strategies of larger burrs since they are easy to advance to the lesions or adjunctive therapy with stents are applicable.[68] The LAO caudal view is an exceptionally good view to visualize the left main and the path of ablation.

Guide Catheter

- Select a guide catheter (with sideholes) that is large enough to accommodate the largest anticipated burr.
- Use larger lumen catheters (generally 9 Fr) even with smaller burrs since rotating in or near the guide catheter may sometimes be necessary.

Guidewire

- The Type C guidewire is generally used.
- Selection of the artery for guidewire placement in the left anterior descending or circumflex may allow preferential or "directional" rotational atherectomy (see Figure 3.15, page 66) of the protected left main.

Burr Selection

- A stepped-burr approach is recommended.
- Large burrs or adjunctive therapy may be required.
- If rotastent is considered, lesion compliance may be assessed after each burr with PTCA at 8 atm to assure that full stent expansion is achievable (see Chapter 6 "Rotastent", on page 224).

Ablation Technique

- Use gentle advancement avoiding decelerations greater than 5,000 rpm with ablation times of 15–30 sec./run.
- It may be difficult to get a "true platform speed" when activating in the guide catheter.
- Coaxiality is essential in platforming within the guide catheter.

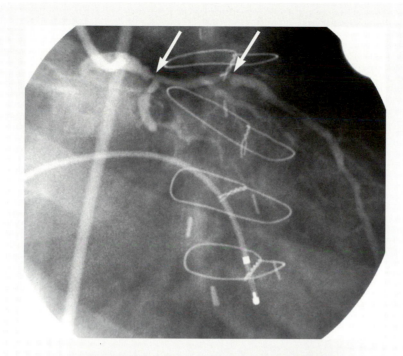

Figure 4.6 A&B

Protected Left Main Artery

Case Information:
- Guide Catheter: 9 Fr JL-4
- Guidewire: Type C
- Pacemaker: Yes
- Burrs: 1.5, 2.0, 2.15 mm
- PTCA: 3.5 x 20 mm
  @ 1 atm

A) This 62 year-old male had bypass surgery eight years prior with intact grafts to the circumflex and RCA but with increasing angina. An 80% occlusion of the left main and a 90% stenosis of the LAD were noted (arrows).

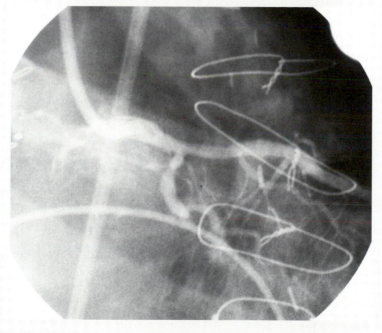

B) The lesions were treated with primary therapy using 1.5, 2.0 and 2.15 mm burrs followed by PTCA at low pressure.

- Exit the guide catheter with a gentle forward motion since the device may "jump" when transitioning to the coronary artery.
- It is often necessary to disengage the guide catheter in left main disease to completely ablate the lesion.
- Frequent runs across the stenosis are recommended especially in discrete disease since the burr may "slip" by the lesion.

Strategy

- Due to the large vessel size adjunctive therapy such as rotastent is often used.
- Directional rotational atherectomy using favorable guidewire bias can be performed in protected left main disease since the guidewire can be placed in the circumflex or the LAD, thereby altering the cutting orientation (see Figure 3.15, page 66).

Figure 4.7 A-C

Protected LMCA

Case Information:
- Guide Catheter: 9 Fr AL-1.5 with sideholes
- Guidewire: Traverse exchanged for a Type C
- Pacemaker: Yes
- Burrs: 1.25, 1.5, 2.15 mm
- PTCA: 3.5 x 30 mm @ 4 atm, 3.0 x 30 mm @ 2.5 atm

A) This 59 year-old man, who was 6 years post-bypass surgery, returned with recurrent angina. The distal left main and distal circumflex had severe lesions.

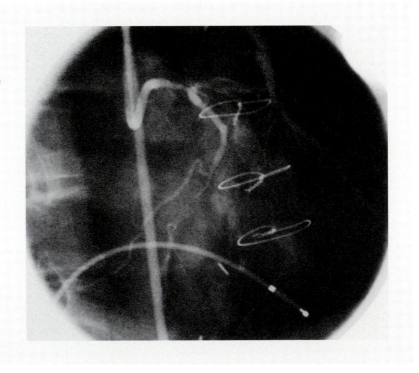

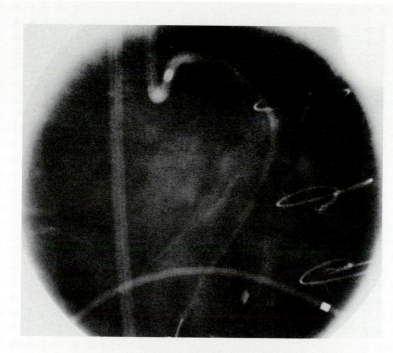

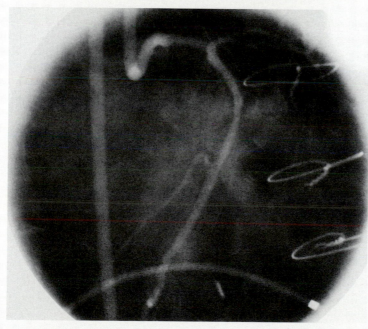

Figure 4.7 B&C
continued

B) The distal left main was treated with a 1.25, 1.5 and 2.15 mm burrs. The 2.15 mm burr was too large to treat the lesion in the distal circumflex.

C) PTCA, using a 3.0 mm balloon at 2.5 atm. in the circumflex and a 3.5 mm balloon at 4 atm. in the left main, resulted in a minimum residual stenosis and excellent flow.

Saphenous Vein Grafts

The Rotablator system is not used in the body of saphenous vein grafts due to the soft elastic morphology of these lesions. The anastomosis of the graft to the native vessel is the site that has received the most attention.[69] The anastomosis site is typically a fibrotic segment. Although little data has been accumulated on the use of rotational atherectomy in the aorto-ostial location of vein grafts,[70] this lesion may benefit from debulking.

Guide Catheter

- Select a guide catheter (with sideholes) that is large enough to accommodate the largest anticipated burr.
- A 90 cm guide catheter may be needed for very distal lesions.
- Guide catheter support for the distal anastomotic lesions is important since the burr is advanced through the saphenous vein graft nonactivated.

Guidewire

- A Type C or a RotaWire Extra Support wire is recommended to assist in nonactivated advancement through the vein graft.

Burr Selection

- A stepped-burr approach is advocated in these lesions.
- Due to the fibrotic nature of these lesions, larger burr-to-artery ratios may be needed (0.7–0.8) to achieve increased lesion compliance (Figure 3.22, page 81).

Ablation Technique

- Use gentle advancement avoiding decelerations greater than 5,000 rpm and keep ablation times to 15–30 sec./run.
- Flow in vein grafts can be slow, especially in the grafts that are patchoulis. Therefore, short ablation runs should be used.

Strategy

- The platform segment should be as near to the lesion as possible in order to avoid agitating any soft plaque in the vein graft.
- If slow flow develops, especially if due to debris from the vein graft, verapamil (approximately 100–150 µg) can be beneficial.

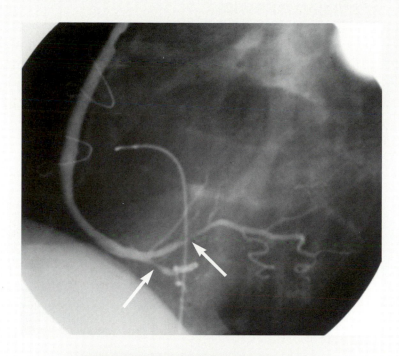

Figure 4.8 A&B

SVG Anastomosis

Case Information:
- Guide Catheter: 9 Fr JR-4
- Guidewire: Type A
- Pacemaker: Yes
- Burrs: 1.5, 1.75 mm
- PTCA: 3.0 x 30 mm @ 4 atm

A) This 65 year-old man was 20 years post-triple-vessel bypass surgery and presented with recurrent angina. Because of possible thrombus within the graft, the patient was treated with coumadin for 1 month prior to atherectomy of the anastomosis of the PDA and a lesion in the adjacent LV extension branch (arrows). The LV extension branch was treated first with a 1.5 mm burr followed by a 3.0 mm balloon at 1 atm. The balloon did not fully open so a 1.75 mm burr was used followed by a 3.0 mm balloon at 4 atm. (See "Interpolated Angioplasty" on page 106.)

B) The lesion at the anastomosis to the PDA was crossed with a HI-Torque Floppy, exchanged for a Type C wire and treated with a 1.75 mm burr followed by the 3.0 mm balloon at 4 atm with the final result shown.

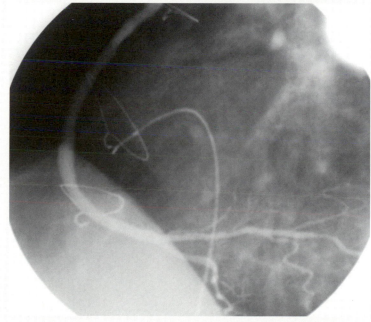

Small Branch Arteries

The use of rotational atherectomy in small branch vessels such as diagonals and obtuse marginals has an important role in revascularization. Often the disease in these vessels occurs as the branch is given off from the major epicardial vessel, and is angulated and poorly responsive to PTCA. These lesions require special attention with the Rotablator system.

Guide Catheter

- Select a guide catheter (with sideholes) that is large enough to accommodate the largest anticipated burr.
- Select a guide catheter which maximizes coaxial placement.

Guidewire

- The Type A or RotaWire guidewires may be required due to limited vessel length.
- The flexibility of the RotaWire Floppy and its shorter platinum

Figure 4.9 A&B

Branch Ostial Disease

Case Information:
- Guide Catheter: 9 Fr JL-4
- Guidewire: Type C
- Pacemaker: No
- Burrs: Dx 1.25, 1.5 mm; LAD 1.75, 2.25 mm
- PTCA: 3.5 x 30 mm perfusion (LAD) and 3.0 x 20 mm (Dx)

A) This bifurcation lesion involved the LAD and a severely angulated takeoff at the diagonal. Initial attempts to treat the diagonal with PTCA (8–10 atm) failed.

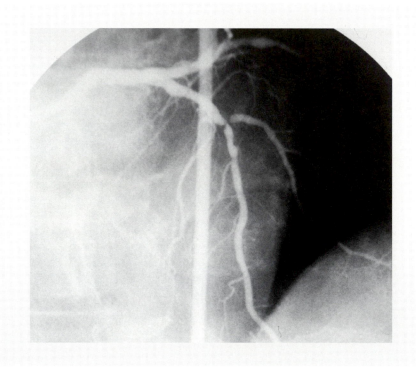

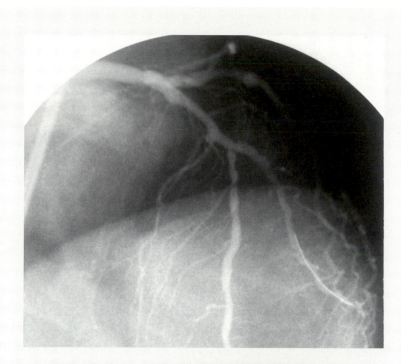

B) Subsequently, the diagonal branch was treated with 1.25 and 1.5 mm burrs. Post-atherectomy, a second guidewire was placed to secure the LAD and a 3.0 mm balloon was inflated at the ostium of the diagonal. The diagonal guidewire was removed and the guidewire in the LAD was exchanged for a Type C. The LAD was treated with 1.75 and 2.25 mm burrs.

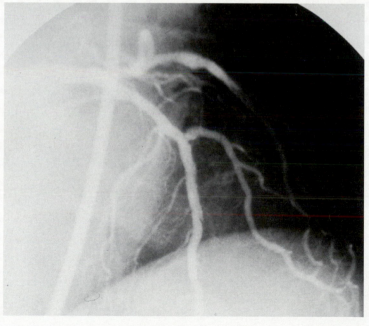

C) Post-atherectomy a protecting guidewire was reinserted into the diagonal and a 3.5 mm perfusion balloon was used to dilate the LAD. Subsequently, "kissing" balloons with the 3.0 and 3.5 mm balloons were used to complete the procedure with the final result shown.

These multiple guidewire exchanges were necessary since double-wire techniques are not possible during atherectomy as the wire would be cut by the rotating burr.

tip may facilitate treatment in tortuous or angulated vessels with a short distal bed.

Burr Selection

- A stepped-burr approach is recommended.
- Undersizing the burrs in small vessels is recommended, especially with branch ostial disease, due to the prevalence of severe angulation and guidewire bias. Tortuosity in small vessels with guidewire bias may result in perforation even with burr-to-artery ratios in the 0.6–0.7 range (see Chapter 7, "Perforations", page 254).
- Careful assessment of luminal gains after each burr may reveal a larger-than-expected gain due to guidewire bias.

Ablation Technique

- Use gentle advancement avoiding decelerations greater than 5,000 rpm and keep ablation times to 15–30 sec./run.
- In severely angulated lesions a "pecking" approach may reduce the incidence of perforation. This is due to a limited time sustained at one point for the burr to ablate radially.
- With small runoff beds, limit ablation runs to approximately 15 seconds and retract burr sufficiently to permit flow between ablation runs.

Strategy

- Treatment of a branch off a larger epicardial vessel will leave the larger conduit unprotected. This is acceptable once it is assumed that even with vasospasm or minimal plaque shifting it will be easy to place a guidewire in the unprotected vessel.
- Lesion modification is almost the rule in branch ostial disease. The compliance change after debulking with a small burr is often significant and allows a balloon to be fully inflated at low pressures. Generally, use a burr-to-artery ratio of approximately 0.6 for lesion modification.

Treatment of Multiple Vessels

The primary concern in the treatment of multiple vessels with rotational atherectomy, is the left ventricular function. Transient left ventricular dysfunction is not unusual during the Rotablator procedure, especially in lesions with excessive plaque burden. The impact of this dysfunction is correlated with the amount of myocardium subtended by the vessel. Therefore, it is advisable to treat vessels that each independently serve large territories in a staged design. If one of the lesions is located in a secondary or a small branch, then treating both vessels during the same procedure is reasonable.

The use of PTCA in one vessel and the Rotablator system in the other should be predicated on the result of the first lesion and the patient's clinical and hemodynamic status. Hypotension following treatment with the Rotablator system is not uncommon, and can be attributed to vasospasm or administration of large amounts of vasodilators and can adversely affect a vessel that was previously treated in the same procedure.

Treatment by Lesion Location

Chapter 5

Lesion location is a significant factor in treating coronary artery disease with rotational atherectomy. This section is designed as a reference to highlight the major considerations in each lesion location.

Proximal Lesions

Proximal lesions are often located in segments with large reference diameters, and are, therefore, associated with larger burrs. This is important to consider when selecting guide catheters in this lesion type. When placing the guide catheter, attempt to center the guidewire as much as possible to reduce the effects of unfavorable guidewire bias. Treatment in proximal lesions requires similar technical skills to those discussed in treating ostial lesions.

Guide Catheter:
- Select a guide catheter (with sideholes) that is large enough to accommodate the largest anticipated burr.
- The guide catheter needs to be coaxial.
- Since the cutting vector in the proximal segment is dependent on the guide catheter, selecting one that can be telescoped or deep-seated into the target vessel is advantageous.
- A curve should be selected that does not force the guidewire radially into the wall (see Figure 3.4, page 47).

> **Guide Catheter Suggestion**
> Selecting a guide catheter that can be telescoped or directed toward the target vessel is advantageous.

Guidewire:

- Typically, the Rotablator guidewire is not difficult to pass, unless the entrance into the lesion is severely angulated. The right angle off the left circumflex is one such example.

- Advancing into the distal vessel around significant bends can be difficult since resistance on the guidewire increases as it passes through the proximal lesion which compromises the "pushability".

- The platinum tip should extend beyond the lesion, but not necessarily to the most distal segment of the vessel. Extending the tip distally may place unnecessary radial stress on wall of the vessel (see Figure 3.13, page 162), especially in tortuous vessels. In tortuous vessels, vessel straightening or "pseudolesions" may compromise the outflow of particles, and potentially enhance the vasoreactivity of the vessel. One solution

Figure 5.1 A-C

Proximal LAD

Case Information:
- Guide Catheter: 8 Fr JL-4
- Guidewire: Type C
- Pacemaker: No
- Burrs: 1.25, 1.75 mm
- PTCA: 3.0 x 30 mm
  @ 1 atm

A) This 73 year-old woman developed increasing exertional angina with occasional rest angina and had a 90% stenosis of the proximal LAD (arrow). This heavily calcified 13 mm lesion was treated with 1.25 and 1.75 mm burrs.

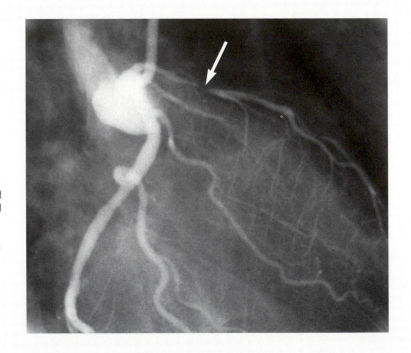

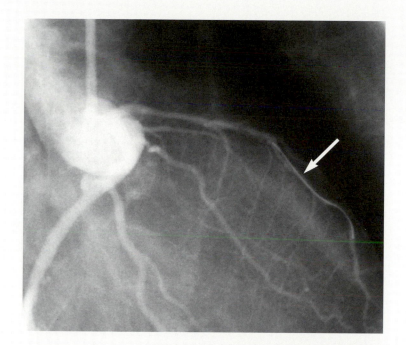

Figure 5.1 B&C
continued

B) In this post-atherectomy view note the proximal location of the guidewire (arrow). This placement results in reduced sideload forces. Poor coaxial alignment of the guide catheter made the burr difficult to advance.

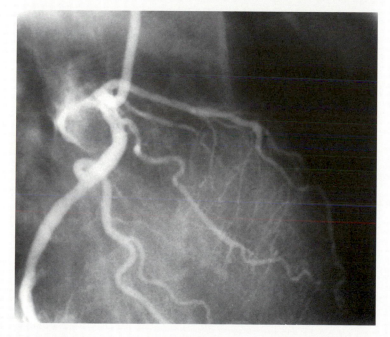

C) Post-atherectomy, the lesion was treated with a 3.0 mm balloon at 1 atm with this final result.

Figure 5.2 A&B

Platforming in Left Main

Case Information:
- Guide Catheter: 8 Fr JL-4
- Guidewire: Type C
- Pacemaker: Yes
- Burrs: 1.5, 2.0 mm
- PTCA: 3.0 x 30 mm
  @ 6 atm

A) This long lesion of the LAD ostium and the diagonal takeoff was treated with 1.5 and 2.0 mm burrs. Platforming in the left main was necessary.

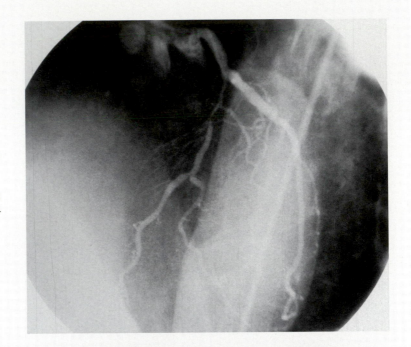

B) Post-atherectomy, there was slow flow or vasospasm in the diagonal. Intervention in the diagonal was not performed since the patient was pain free and without ECG changes. Adjunctive PTCA was used in the LAD.

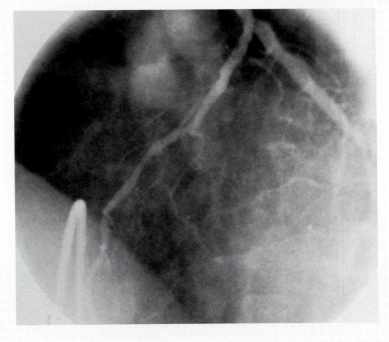

is to avoid anchoring the guidewire in the distal limits of the vessel (Figure 5.1).

Pacemaker:
- The use of larger burrs, especially when platforming in the left main, can cause heart block. Consequently, a temporary pacing wire should be placed when treating these vessels.

Burr Selection:
- A stepped-burr approach is recommended.
- Lesions should always be closely interrogated after each burr prior to going to larger devices since the lumens achieved may actually exceed the size of the burr used due to guidewire bias.
- Prior to activating larger burrs, confirm that there is flow around the device in the platform segment. Often the "normal" reference segment can be deceptive and the burr may need to be withdrawn further proximally, occasionally into the left main (Figure 5.2).

Ablation Technique:
- Use gentle advancement avoiding decelerations greater than 5,000 rpm and keep ablation times to 15–30 sec./run.
- Ablation should follow the techniques outlined in methods based on lesion morphology (Chapter 6).
- Vasodilators should be used generously to prevent spasm of the septals and diagonals in the left circulation or the right ventricular branches when treating the proximal RCA.

Strategy:
- An integrated strategy (device synergy) is sometimes performed in proximal lesions, since they often occur in larger segments.
- Attempt to debulk with the Rotablator system to achieve a 0.70–0.85 burr-to-artery ratio, and then use adjunctive PTCA, stent or DCA if required.

Distal Lesions

The successful treatment of distal lesions relies principally on vessel characteristics proximally and the morphology of the lesion. In tortuous or rigid vessels, it may be difficult to advance the guidewire and larger burrs to the lesion site (Figure 5.3).

Guide Catheter:

- Select a guide catheter (with sideholes) that is large enough to accommodate the largest anticipated burr.
- Conventional shapes with an emphasis on support, are recommended.
- A guide catheter that is not coaxial to the vessel will increase the difficulty in advancing a nonactivated burr to the lesion. Repositioning the guide catheter coaxially in the vessel may allow transmission of the force along the guidewire permitting the burr to advance more easily.
- Frequently, activated advancement techniques are required.

Guidewire:

- The guidewire may be difficult to negotiate in tortuous, rigid or inelastic vessels even in areas without significant stenosis.
- Opting for conventional guidewire systems and exchanging for the Rotablator guidewire may facilitate and expedite the procedure.
- Since the distal vessel beyond the lesion may be limited in length, the wires with a shorter platinum tips, like the Type A or RotaWire guidewires can be used instead of the Type C guidewire (Figure 5.4).
- The position of the guidewire should always be assessed to ensure it has not entered a small branch. This position can be confirmed by flow beyond the tip of the guidewire.
- The RotaWire Floppy guidewire with its greater flexibility and shorter tip may ease guidewire placement in most vessels. Occasionally this flexibility may not provide adequate support

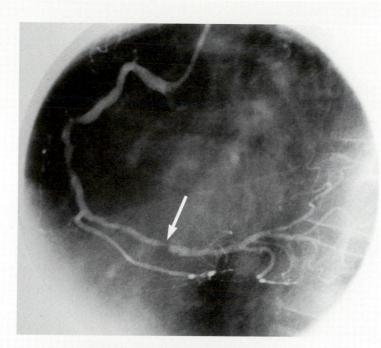

Figure 5.3 A&B

Burr Advancement to a Distal Lesion

Case Information:
- Guide Catheter: 8 Fr Hockeystick
- Guidewire: Type C
- Pacemaker: Yes
- Burrs: 1.5 mm
- PTCA: 3.0 x 30 mm @ 6 atm

A) Baseline angiography revealed a severely calcified, inelastic and tortuous RCA. A 1.5 mm burr required high-speed advancement to reach the distal lesion (arrow).

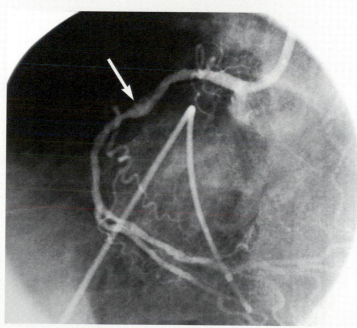

B) Activated advancement of the burr from just beyond the guide catheter resulted in ablation of inelastic tissue. Haziness in the mid-segment of the vessel (arrow) with a "guttering effect" on the outside border is observed. Because of the guidewire tension against the wall, burrs larger than 1.5 mm were not used. The distal lesion was dilated post-atherectomy with a 3.0 mm balloon at 6 atm with the result shown here.

to advance the burr in inelastic, tortuous vessels (see Figure 3.23). Exchanging for the RotaWire Extra Support may be beneficial.

Burr Selection:
- A stepped-burr approach is recommended.
- Burr sizing should follow standard techniques.
- Tortuosity, rigidity or moderate disease in the proximal and mid-segment of the vessel may limit the advancement of larger burrs into distal lesions (Figure 5.3).
- If the burr cannot be advanced non-activated, the burr can be advanced at either high or preferably low speed. (See Chapter 3 "Burr Advancement", page 82.)
- When using a "tapping technique", release tension on the driveshaft as described in Chapter 3, "Relief of Driveshaft Tension", page 86, prior to activation.

Ablation Technique:
- Use gentle advancement avoiding decelerations greater than 5,000 rpm and keep ablation times to 15–30 sec./run.
- Since distal vessels often have limited runoff, use shorter runs (< 30 seconds) with longer intervals between ablations.
- Retract the burr to a proximal position to assure adequate antegrade flow during intervals between ablation.
- Attempt to advance the driveshaft system as close to the lesion as possible to avoid having a fully protracted system.

Strategy:
- Minimal debulking followed by adjunctive PTCA may be advisable, since larger burrs can be difficult to position distally. If the lesion is accessible for large burrs, standard strategy is performed.
- In distal vessels, tapering can be significant and care must be taken when advancing larger burrs into these smaller vessels, to avoid perforation. Frequent contrast injections are helpful (see Figure 3.29, page 94).

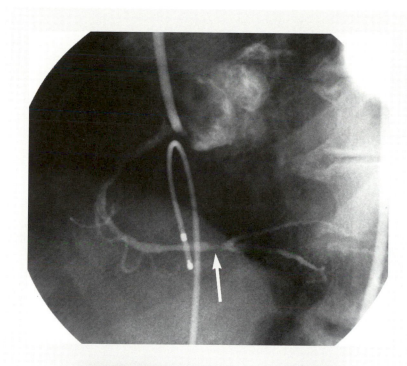

Figure 5.4 A&B

**Proximal and Distal
RCA Lesions**

Case Information:
- Guide Catheter: 9 Fr JR-4
- Guidewire: Type A
- Pacemaker: Yes
- Burrs: 1.25, 1.75 mm
- PTCA: 3.0 mm x 20 mm
  distal
- DCA: 7 Fr in proximal
  lesion

A) This pretreatment
angiogram shows a long
proximal right coronary lesion
and a distal lesion just prior to
the bifurcation (arrow). The
shorter tipped Type A
guidewire was used due to
the limited length beyond the
distal lesion.

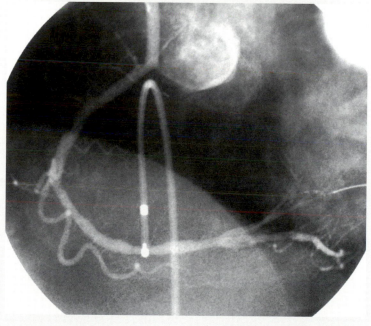

B) After treatment of the
proximal and distal lesions
with 1.25 and 1.75 mm burrs
the distal lesion was treated
with a 3.0 mm balloon at
2 atm and the proximal lesion
was treated with DCA.

Multiple Lesions in a Single Vessel (Diffuse Disease)

Multiple lesions in a single vessel are challenging cases. These lesions can require the use of a combination of multiple burrs and balloons. Although predilation at the most distal lesion to improve outflow might be considered, the recommendation is generally not to predilate a distal lesion, especially if the lesion is amenable to treatment with rotational atherectomy; rather, ablate the lesions and subsequently assess the strategy.

Guide Catheter:

- Select a guide catheter (with sideholes) that is large enough to accommodate the largest anticipated burr.
- Good support is often required in these lesion subtypes.

Figure 5.5 A-C

Segmental Ablation

Case Information:
- Guide Catheter: 8 Fr JR-4
- Guidewire: Type C
- Pacemaker: Yes
- Burrs: 1.5, 1.75 mm
- PTCA: 3.0 x 30 mm
  @ 4 atm

A) The LAO projection shows a long diffusely diseased RCA with multiple lesions.

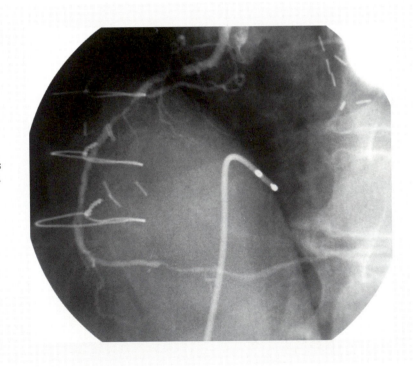

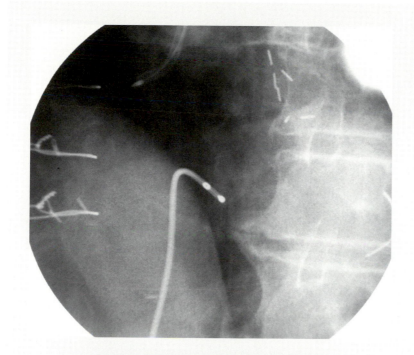

Figure 5.5 B&C
continued

B) The burr was positioned just distal to the guide catheter in the platform segment and the artery was treated with 1.5 and 1.75 mm burrs. Segmental ablation runs were performed for 15–30 seconds each.

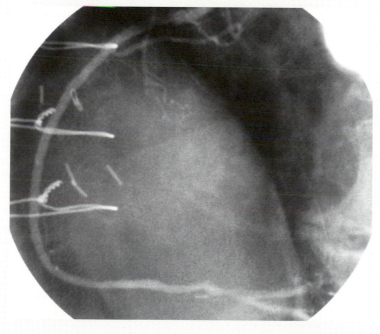

C) After PTCA with a 3.0 mm balloon at 4 atm., there was minimal residual stenosis.

Guidewire:

- Depending on lesion morphology, the Type C or RotaWire Floppy guidewire, can be used, although the use of conventional wires initially, and exchanging for the Rotablator guidewire can, in complex vessels, be the quickest and easiest method.
- If the distal lesion is approaching the terminus of the epicardial vessel, the Type A or RotaWire guidewire may be required, due to the shorter platinum tip.

Burr Selection:

- A stepped-burr approach is recommended.
- In a vessel with multiple lesions, the most distal lesion determines the initial burr size.
- In tapering vessels, note landmarks and burr size since advancing oversized burrs in small distal vessels can result in perforation (see Figure 3.29, page 94).
- If there is angiographic or clinical compromise after treatment, low-pressure PTCA should be used prior to stepping up to larger burrs (see Chapter 3, "Interpolated Angioplasty", page 106).

Ablation Technique:

- Use gentle advancement avoiding decelerations greater than 5,000 rpm and keep ablation times to 15–30 sec./run. The interval between the runs should be long enough to permit stabilization of the electrocardiogram and hemodynamics.
- Do not try to achieve a lumen "as fast as possible" in these cases.
- Segmental ablations are recommended.
- Frequent contrast injections are needed if there is an abrupt decrease in vessel size distally.

Strategy:

- A strategy of either primary therapy or lesion modification can often be used depending on the overall lesion morphology and patient's tolerance after the burr treatment.

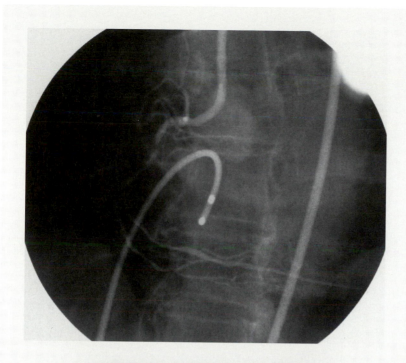

Figure 5.6 A&B

Diffuse Disease

Case Information:
- Guide Catheter: 8 Fr JR-3.5
- Guidewire: Type C
- Pacemaker: Yes
- Burrs: 1.25, 1.5, 1.75 mm
- PTCA: 2.5 x 30 mm
  @ 4 atm

A) This 55 year-old male presented with increasing angina and a 95% occlusion of the proximal RCA with diffuse disease extending to the PDA.

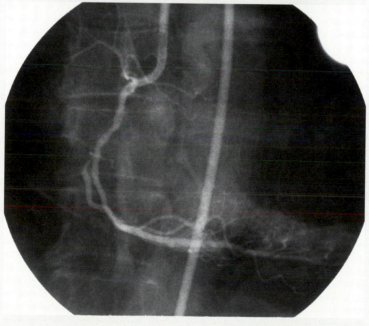

B) Because the vessel was small and the lesion was long, rotational atherectomy was initiated using a 1.25 mm burr. This was followed by 1.5 and 1.75 mm burrs. PTCA with a 2.5 mm balloon at 4 atm gave this final result.

Figure 5.7 A-C

Access via SVG

Case Information:
- Guide Catheter: 8 Fr JR-4
- Guidewire: Type C
- Pacemaker: No
- Burrs: 1.25 mm
- PTCA: 1.5 x 30 mm
  @ 10 atm; 2.0 x 30 mm
  @ 8 atm; 2.5 x 30
  @ 4 atm.

A) This 61 year-old diabetic, hypertensive female with a history of bypass surgery 9 years prior and an ejection fraction of < 30% was treated for her diffusely diseased LAD through the widely patent saphenous vein graft.

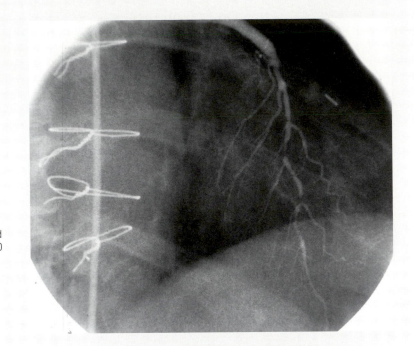

B) The proximal and mid segments of the LAD were treated with a 1.25 mm burr followed by a 2.0 mm balloon inflated to 5.5 atm. The guidewire was then advanced and the distal vessel was treated with the 1.25 mm burr and a 1.5 mm balloon at 10 atm.

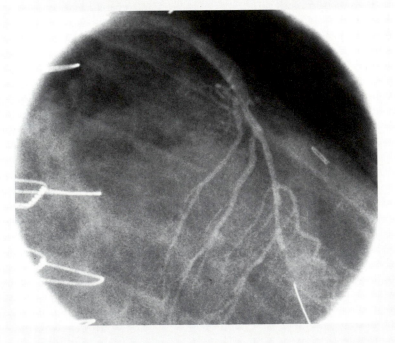

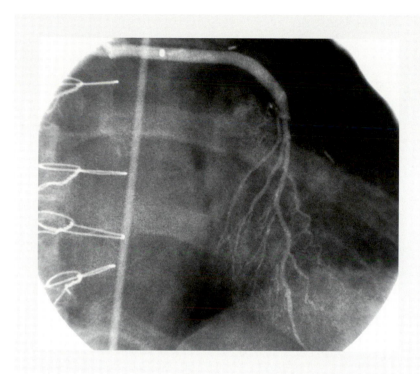

Figure 5.7 C
continued

C) Following completion of the distal segment the proximal and mid-segments were again dilated using 2.0 and 2.5 mm balloons with this final result.

- Vasospasm distally may compromise runoff. In this case, low-pressure PTCA and further rotational atherectomy can be applied.

- If the proximal lesions need more debulking, performing adjunctive PTCA distally to improve flow may permit the use of larger burrs proximally.

- Treatment of multiple lesions in a single vessel may be complicated by an advancer knob limit. When fully advanced, the knob may not allow the device to reach the most distal lesions. A useful technique for this morphology is to park the burr distal to the previously treated lesions and then advance the catheter, situating the burr in a platform segment proximal to the next lesion intended for treatment. The burr can be positioned distally, using a nonactivated or activated low-speed advancement technique. (See Chapter 3, "Burr Advancement", page 82.)

Ostial Lesions*

The frequent fibrocalcific characteristics of these lesions make them well suited for this technology. Although not an FDA approved indication, several reports document good outcome in these lesions.[40,41,42]

Guide Catheter:

- Select a guide catheter (with sideholes) that is large enough to accommodate the largest anticipated burr.
- The key to successful treatment of aorto-ostial lesions is guide catheter selection. A guide should be chosen that can achieve coaxial placement. A coaxial guide that is not intubated is preferred to one that is intubated in the ostium but not well aligned. These positioning issues can frequently be best appreciated in the RAO projection.
- Certain guide catheters have an advantage. In the aorto-ostial RCA, the hockey-stick shape is often a good choice. In ostial circumflex lesions, especially those with short left main arteries, the Amplatz or a shape that can telescope the guide coaxially into the circumflex are beneficial.
- The straight alignment of the guide catheter is essential in order to center the guidewire (Figure 5.8). A tangentially aligned guide catheter, will alter the position of the guidewire, and may force the burr preferentially to one side of the vessel (guidewire bias).
- In general, the guide catheter should be oversized as it may be necessary to platform the burr within it. While this is not recommended, it may be required due to the often tenuous placement of the guide catheter in the ostium.
- Stiff-tipped guide catheters may be advantageous since softer tipped guides often "fish mouth" and can make it difficult to exit the burr from the guide catheter (Figure 5.9).

Guidewire:

- Type C or RotaWire Floppy guidewires can, in most cases, cross ostial lesions. If after a few attempts it does not move distally in

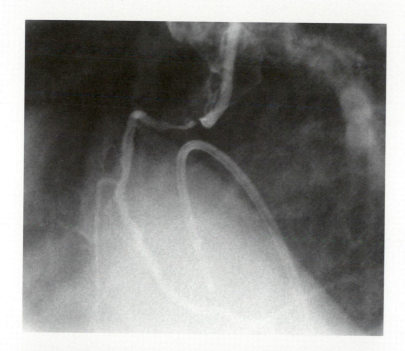

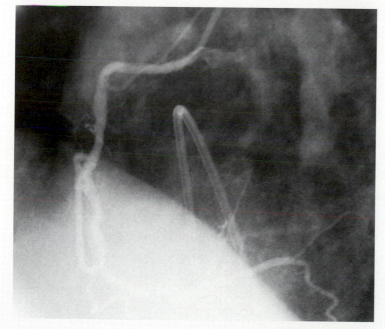

Figure 5.8 A&B

**Aorto-Ostial Disease:
Coaxial Guide Catheter
Alignment**

Case Information:
- Guide Catheter: 9 Fr JR-4
- Guidewire: Type C
- Pacemaker: Yes
- Burrs: 1.5, 2.0 mm
- PTCA: 3.5 mm x 30 mm
  @ 1.5 atm.

A) This 66 year-old male had
a heavily calcified 90%
stenosis of the RCA. In this
pretreatment view, the guide
catheter is coaxial; the
guidewire is placed in the mid
segment creating a coaxial
trajectory of the guidewire.
A 9 Fr guide catheter was
selected to allow for
platforming inside the
catheter. This patient
experienced transient asystole
during ablation, emphasizing
the need for a pacemaker
when treating the RCA,
especially the ostium.

B) Coaxial alignment of the
guide catheter and guidewire
facilitated an excellent
angiographic result.

*Treatment of aorto-ostial
lesions is not an FDA-approved
indication.*

Figure 5.9 A-C

Aorto-Ostial RCA

Case Information:
- Guide Catheter: 9 Fr JR-4
- Guidewire: Type C
- Pacemaker: Yes
- Burrs: 1.25,1.5, 1.75 mm
- PTCA: 4.0 x 20 mm
  @ 6 atm.
- Prophylactic intra-aortic
  balloon pump

A) This LAO projection shows the aorto-ostial lesion* of the RCA. Due to a 20% ejection fraction, the woman was placed on a balloon pump prophylactically.

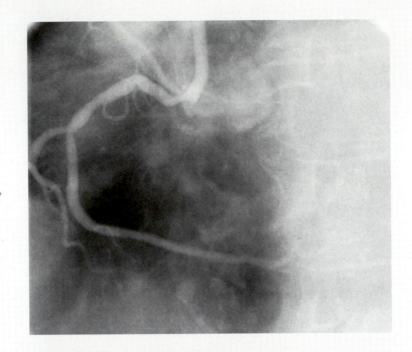

B) Note the accentuation of the ostial lesion and the pseudolesion in the proximal RCA (arrow) formed by guidewire tension. In the presence of the vessel deformity by the guidewire tangential ablation may result and a strategy of lesion modification is recommended. Maintaining the guidewire in a more proximal position may have been advantageous in this case (the spring tip is visible just proximal to the bifurcation).

*Treatment of aorto-ostial lesions is not an FDA-approved indication.

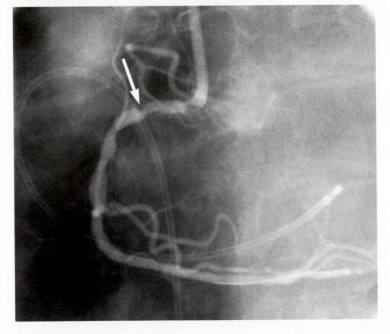

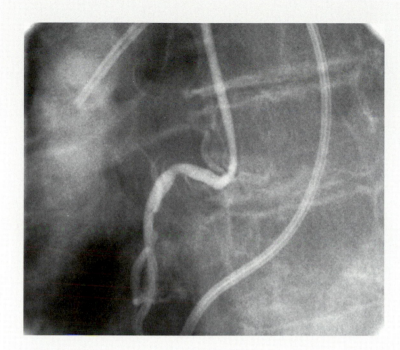

Figure 5.9 C
continued

C) After rotational atherectomy with 1.25, 1.5, and 1.75 mm burrs and PTCA with a 4.0 mm balloon at 6 atm., the aorto-ostial lesion has minimal residual stenosis. The pseudolesions seen in (B) had been relieved by the removal of the guidewire.

the vessel because it has been "trapped" in the lesion, switch to a conventional PTCA wire and exchange for the Rotablator guidewire.

- Advancing the guidewire into the most distal segment of the vessel is not necessary. In fact, it may improve guidewire "centering" (minimizing guidewire bias) if the tip is left just beyond the lesion.
- The lie of the guidewire is essential in ostial lesions since the positioning will impact burr sizing (Figures 5.8 and 5.9).

Pacemaker:

- A temporary pacemaker should be used when treating ostial RCA, ostial LAD and ostial circumflex disease, since complete heart block can occur with these lesions.

Figure 5.10 A-C

Branch Ostial Lesion

Case Information:
- Guide Catheter: 8 Fr JL-4
- Guidewire: Type C
- Pacemaker: No
- Burrs: 1.25,1.5 mm
- PTCA: 2.5 x 30 mm
  @ 3 atm.

A) This 77 year-old female was treated for a diffuse 45 mm stenosis of the LAD originating near the ostium of the diagonal (arrow).

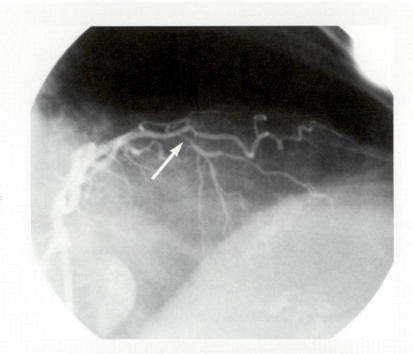

B) The lesion is more apparent in the LAO view (arrow).

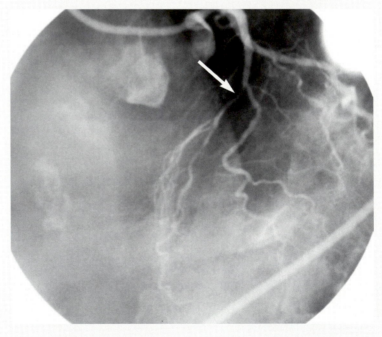

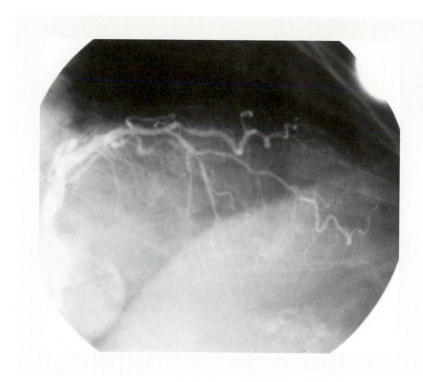

Figure 5.10 C
continued

C) The lesion was treated with 1.25 and 1.5 mm burrs followed by a 2.5 mm balloon at 3 atm.

Burr Selection:

- A stepped-burr approach is recommended.
- Several burrs may be required. Using as many as three burrs in aorto-ostial disease is not infrequent.
- When the guide catheter is vectoring the guidewire to lie tangentially, undersize the initial burr and carefully assess gains after each burr.
- In branch ostial disease (obtuse marginal and diagonal), start with smaller initial burrs (a burr-to-artery ratio of no more than 0.5). Guidewire bias in these often angulated branch points substantially increases the risk of perforation.[64]
- Performing low-pressure PTCA in angled branches is often helpful to assess the gains achieved after the ablation prior to stepping up to larger burrs.

Ablation Technique:

- Use gentle advancement avoiding decelerations greater than 5,000 rpm and keeping ablation times to 15–30 sec./run.
- In aortal-ostial disease, activation of the burr can occur outside the guide catheter, with the burr juxtaposed to the ostium. This position can generally be achieved by advancing the burr while the guide catheter "kicks out of the lesion". If this position cannot be achieved, activation of the burr in the guide catheter may be required.
- Several gentle passes through the lesion are important to ensure that the burr has adequately debulked the lesion. Aorto-ostial lesions are easy to Dotter through or "slip past".
- In the treatment of the ostial LAD and the circumflex, the burr will be platformed in the left main coronary artery. While this practice has not resulted in increased complications, it is advisable not to spend excessive time adjusting the rpm in the left main.
- With severe branch ostial angulation "chipping" or pecking at the lesion is recommended to reduce radial cutting (see Chapter 6, "Angulated Lesions", page 168).

Strategy:

- Primary therapy or lesion modification can be performed in aorto-ostial lesions.
- With branch ostial disease on severe angles, a burr-to-artery ratio of 0.5–0.6 should not be exceeded (generally unfavorable guidewire bias). Adjunctive PTCA is recommended in these cases (lesion modification).
- Determine whether to use adjunctive PTCA, DCA, or stents when the vessel is large or when a larger burr cannot be used due to the angle between the guide and the lesion.
- Interpolated angioplasty is helpful in angulated branch ostial disease (see Chapter 3, "Interpolated Angioplasty", page 106).

Collateralized Vessels

Although one would expect collateralized vessels to impede antegrade flow and particle clearance, this occurrence has not been realized in clinical practice. Collaterals have not been independently correlated with an increased incidence of slow flow and no reflow.

- Burr selection should not be altered by the presence of collaterals.
- The target vessel is often occluded or suboccluded. The strategy should be dictated by those anatomical considerations.
- Diffuse spasm may occur after ablation. It can be difficult to adequately opacify the treatment site in the presence of significant retrograde flow. Administration of nitroglycerin and more robust injections of contrast often solves this problem.
- Low-pressure PTCA between burrs (see Chapter 3, "Interpolated PTCA", page 106) is often helpful in relieving spasm.
- With the reconstitution of antegrade flow, ventricular ectopy is noted occasionally.

Treatment by Lesion Morphology

Chapter 6

The majority of lesion morphologies can be treated with rotational atherectomy (see Table 2.3, page 29). This section provides an analysis of treatment of various lesion morphologies with a critical assessment of techniques used and an emphasis on avoiding potential problems that can emerge during the procedure.

Focal (Discrete) Lesions

Focal or discrete lesions (≤ 10.0 mm) can be treated effectively with the Rotablator procedure. The focal nature of the lesion should not necessarily dictate a single large-burr approach.

Guide Catheter:
- Select a guide catheter (with sideholes) that is large enough to accommodate the largest anticipated burr.

Guidewire:
- The majority of these lesions can be crossed with a Type C or RotaWire Floppy guidewire.
- Type C or RotaWire Extra Support guidewires may be beneficial since the stiffness may improve plaque engagement in discrete lesions. The RotaWire Floppy guidewire should be used if there is significant distal tortuosity.

Figure 6.1 A&B

Focal Lesion of the LAD

Case Information:
- Guide Catheter: 9 Fr JL-4
- Guidewire: Type C
- Pacemaker: No
- Burrs: 1.5, 2.0, 2.15 mm
- PTCA: 3.5 x 20 mm
  @ 1 atm

A) This 68 year-old male presented with new onset exertional angina and an 80% 6 mm LAD lesion (arrow). The lesion was treated with 1.5, 2.0 and 2.15 mm burrs.

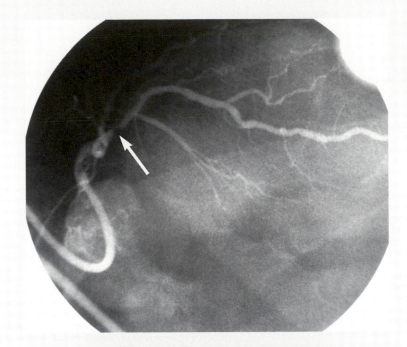

B) After atherectomy and a 3.5 mm balloon at 1 atm. there was no residual stenosis.

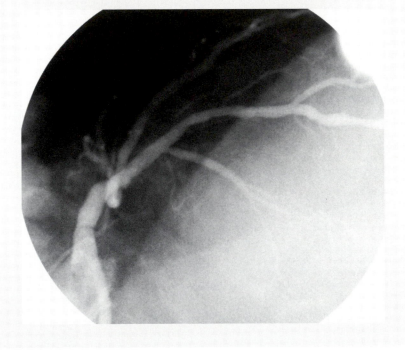

Burr Selection:

- The stepped-burr approach is recommended specifically at focal lesions with significant angulations at branch ostial locations, such as diagonal and obtuse marginal branches. In discrete lesions in straight segments, the largest anticipated burr can be used as a single device, but is discouraged.
- A focal lesion on a severe angle, such as at the ostium of the diagonal or obtuse marginal branch, has been the most frequent site for perforations (see Chapter 7 on "Perforations" page 254).[64, 81] Perforations can often be attributed to the use of oversized burrs on severe angles with guidewire bias. In cases with guidewire bias, oversized burrs can be those with burr-to-artery ratios exceeding 0.6.

Ablation Technique:

- Use gentle advancement avoiding decelerations greater than 5,000 rpm and keep ablation times to 15–30 sec./run.
- The burr has a tendency to "watermelon seed" or slip through the lesion. Adequate ablation can be confirmed by making several slow passes back and forth across the lesion.
- In lesions that are not severely angulated, standard ablation technique can be applied.
- Severely angulated focal lesions at the ostium or branch ostial locations present significant difficulties when ablating. In this situation, pecking or chipping at the lesion is advisable.

Strategy:

- For most discrete lesions, primary therapy can often be achieved.
- In focal lesions on straight or slightly angulated segments, the burr-to-artery ratio is recommended at 0.7–0.9 (primary therapy).
- In segments with severe angulation, the burr-to-artery ratio should not exceed 0.6–0.7 and should be followed by systematic PTCA (lesion modification).

Angulated Lesions

Significantly angulated (> 45°) lesions pose a challenge for rotational atherectomy and should be approached with caution.[50] Guide catheter alignment, guidewire bias, preferential cutting, all require close attention when ablating and selecting burrs in these lesions. Lesion modification is often recommended unless a favorable guidewire bias permits adequate ablation of the plaque mass.

Guide Catheter:

- Select a guide catheter (with sideholes) that is large enough to accommodate the largest anticipated burr.
- Select a guide catheter that centralizes the guidewire to reduce unfavorable guidewire bias, e.g. an Amplatz or Voda catheter for an ostial circumflex lesion.

Guidewire:

- Type C or RotaWire Floppy guidewires are recommended.
- Adjustment of guide catheter for coaxial alignment and placement of the guidewire just beyond the lesion to reduce sidewall tension will minimize tangential vectoring of the guidewire (Figure 3.10, page 56).

Burr Selection:

- A stepped-burr approach is recommended. Incremental steps in burr size should be small in angulated lesions due to the likelihood of the guidewire becoming tangentially oriented and resulting in preferential ablation (Figure 6.4).
- Assess luminal gains after each burr for favorable or unfavorable guidewire bias.
- In severe angles (≥ 60°), undersize the burr and do not attempt to exceed a burr-to-artery ratio of approximately 0.6.
- Maximal debulking should be attempted only if the angle was determined by the plaque and not the native vessel configuration. This can be assessed after ablating with one of the initial burrs.

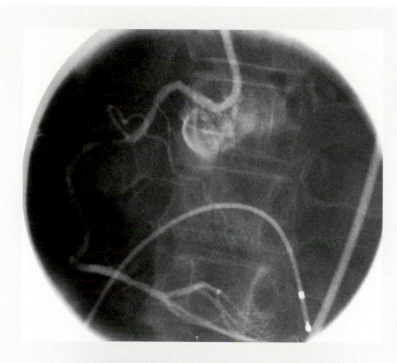

Figure 6.2 A&B

Treatment of Angulated Lesions

Case Information:
- Guide Catheter: 9 Fr Hockeystick
- Guidewire: Type C
- Pacemaker: Yes
- Burrs: 1.5, 2.0 mm
- PTCA: 3.0 x 20 mm @ 4 atm.

A) This LAO view shows the mid right coronary lesion in a serpentine vessel. Due to angulated nature of the vessel, a strategy of lesion modification was chosen. The treatment was started with a 1.5 mm burr, significantly undersized due to the angulation, followed by a 2.0 mm burr and a 3.0 x 20 mm balloon at 4 atm.

B) Post-treatment angiogram with the guidewire in place shows the final result and the straightening of the vessel caused by the guidewire.

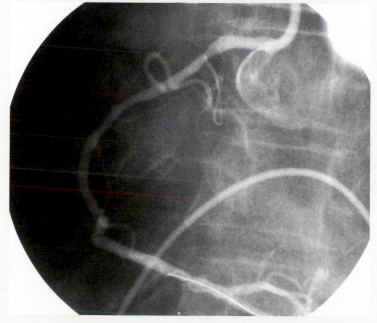

Ablation Technique:

- Use gentle advancement avoiding decelerations greater than 5,000 rpm and keeping ablation times to 15–30 sec./run.
- Ablation technique should permit frequent reassessment with contrast injections to observe the direction of the burr as it tracks through the angulated segment of the lesion.
- A guidewire that "vectors" out of the natural orientation of the angulated vessel may cause preferential ablation and in the worst case, result in perforation (see Figure 7.5, page 256).
- Burr speed may drop due to angulation or curvature in the vessel. To determine whether speed drop is due to a bend or angle, or engagement with the lesion, assess the contrast flow. If contrast passes around the burr when the speed drops, the deceleration is due to the angle, not a lesion. This lower speed, in the bend, becomes the "new" platform speed.
- Ablation in an angulated lesion should use advancing and retracting of the burr exaggerating the oscillating technique towards chipping at the lesion.
- If the device does not cross the lesion due to the severity of the angle, attempt to make larger strokes (pecking technique) with the advancer knob. If this is unsuccessful, use a smaller burr.
- Avoid spinning the burr in a fixed position when treating angulated lesions. The tip of burr may abrade the guidewire and result in a guidewire fracture. Therefore oscillate the burr during treatment and move the guidewire to position a "fresh" segment at the lesions site when multiple runs are used.

Strategy:

- In severe angles use undersized burrs with the objective of increasing the compliance of the vessel.
- Generally do not to exceed a burr-to-artery ratio of 0.6–0.7.
- In most cases, lesion modification is recommended.

Angulated Lesions Graphic Illustrations and Case Studies

The following cases illustrate key issues for angulated lesions.

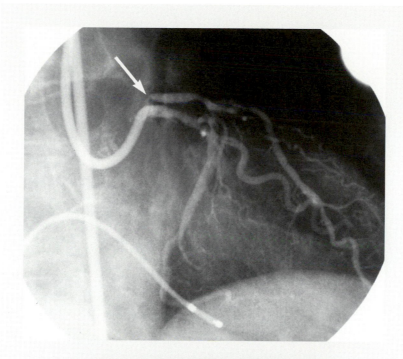

Figure 6.3 A&B

Angulated Lesion Treated with Adjunctive DCA

Case Information:
- Guide Catheter: 10 Fr DVI
- Guidewire: Type C
- Pacemaker: Yes
- Burrs: 1.5, 2.0 mm
- DCA: Yes
- PTCA: 4.0 x 20 mm @ 6 atm.

A) The 90% stenosis of a severely angulated calcified ostial LAD lesion (arrow) was treated with a small burr-to-artery ratio (< 0.6). The lesion was further modified with directional coronary atherectomy.

B) After adjunctive DCA the stenosis was reduced to 20%.

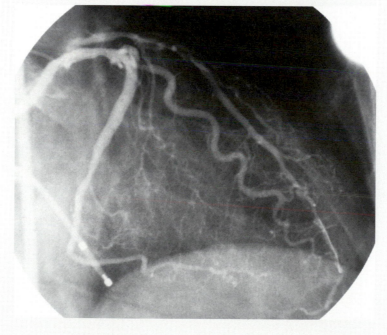

Figure 6.4 A-D

Directional Rotational Atherectomy

Case Information:
- Guide Catheter: 9 Fr AL-2
- Guidewire: Type C
- Pacemaker: Yes
- Burrs: 1.75, 2.15 mm
- PTCA: 3.0 x 30 mm
  @ 2 atm. perfusion

A) This pretreatment RAO projection shows an angulated 80% lesion in the proximal LCx (arrow) and a 70% lesion in the distal circumflex.

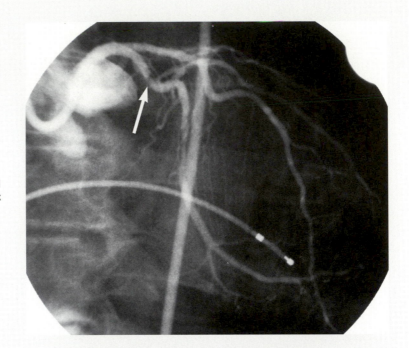

B) This angiogram, taken after treatment of both lesions with a 1.75 mm burr, reveals a better than expected result at the proximal lesion due to guidewire bias to the upper wall of the vessel where the majority of the plaque in this eccentric lesion was most likely positioned.

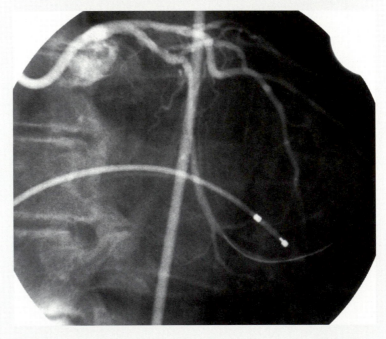

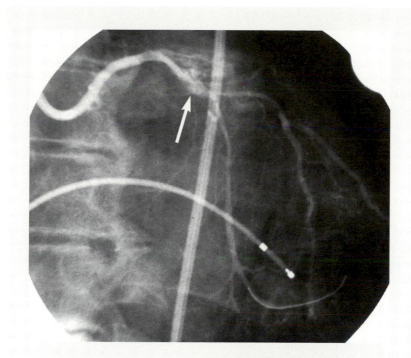

Figure 6.4 C&D
continued

C) When a 2.15 mm burr was used in the proximal lesion, guidewire bias contributed to the perforation (arrow).

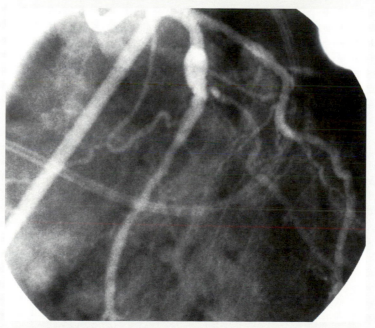

D) After treatment of both proximal and distal lesions with a 3.0 x 30 mm perfusion balloon, the perforation was sealed leaving an aneurysmal appearance at the proximal site and a 20% stenosis distally.

In light of the "excessive" luminal gain achieved with the 1.75 mm burr due to directional rotational atherectomy of the eccentrically located plaque, incremental burr sizes should not have been used.

Bifurcation Lesions

A double-wire technique to protect an adjacent vessel is not possible in bifurcation lesions with the Rotablator system, since a second guidewire would be cut by the diamond chips of the burr. Without a protecting guidewire, spasm, slow flow or plaque shifting can be a threat to the untreated branch. Ideally, only minimal plaque shifting should occur with rotational atherectomy. The lesion within a branch considered most difficult to cross with a guidewire should be considered as the initial treatment site. The types of bifurcation lesions are illustrated in Figure 6.8.

Guide Catheter:
• Select a guide catheter (with sideholes) that is large enough to accommodate the largest anticipated burr.
• The guide catheter should provide adequate support and accommodate two balloons if a "kissing balloon" technique is needed adjunctively.

Guidewire:
• Assess for guidewire bias, especially in branch ostial lesions.
• It is advantageous to initially treat the vessel in which the guidewire placement is anticipated to be most difficult.
• Placing the guidewire in different branches may provide favorable guidewire bias and achieve a larger lumen than the burr size used (Figure 3.15, page 66).

Burr Selection:
• A stepped-burr approach is recommended.
• Burr sizing should follow standard techniques depending on lesion morphology.
• Primary therapy may be preferred since the septum of the bifurcation is not stretched (as with PTCA) and the adjacent lumen should not be compromised.
• A low burr-to-artery ratio (0.5) is recommended in severely angulated branch ostial bifurcation lesions. Often the diagonal ostium off the LAD is the site of such a lesion, as is the obtuse marginal ostium off the circumflex artery.

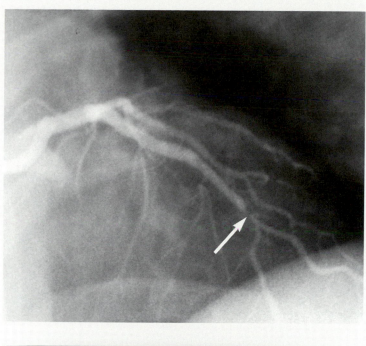

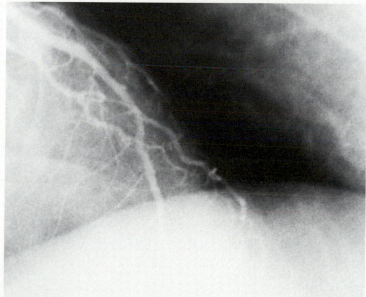

Figure 6.5 A&B

LAD Diagonal Bifurcation

Case Information:
- Guide Catheter: 8 Fr FL-4
- Guidewire: ACS™ Intermediate exchange for Type C
- Pacemaker: No
- Burrs: 1.5 mm
- PTCA: 2 x 2.5 x 30 mm @ 2 atm "kissing"

A) This 37 year-old insulin-dependent diabetic female experienced restenosis of her mid-LAD at the bifurcation with the diagonal (arrow). This represents a Type A bifurcation lesion (Figure 6.8). There was difficulty passing the guidewire into the LAD. After several attempts an intermediate wire was placed and exchanged for the Type C wire. After treatment of the LAD with a 1.5 mm burr, the diagonal experienced spasm and slow flow.

B) The LAD and diagonal were treated with sequential and "kissing" 2.5 mm balloons with a good result and TIMI III flow.

- If it is possible to achieve favorable guidewire bias, larger burrs may not be necessary.

Ablation Technique:
- Use gentle advancement avoiding decelerations greater than 5,000 rpm and keeping ablation times to 15–30 sec./run.
- Standard ablation technique should be applied with occasional contrast injections to judge the status of the non-protected vessel.
- If the branch is angulated, use contrast injections to visualize the path of the burr using broader strokes (pecking technique) when the guidewire lies eccentrically (guidewire bias).
- Use contrast injections to determine if rpm drops are due to angulation, or to the burr engaging the lesion.

Strategy:

Two approaches are possible: 1) Ablate both limbs of the bifurcation, or 2) ablate one and dilate the other. Consider the

Figure 6.6 A-C

Severe Angulation at Point of Trifurcation

Case Information:
- Guide Catheter: 8 Fr JR-4
- Guidewire: Type C
- Pacemaker: Yes
- Burrs: 1.5 mm
- PTCA: 3.0 mm x 20 mm @ 6 atm

A) The LAO projection shows an untreated complex trifurcation lesion (arrow) of the distal RCA (Type D, Figure 6.8).

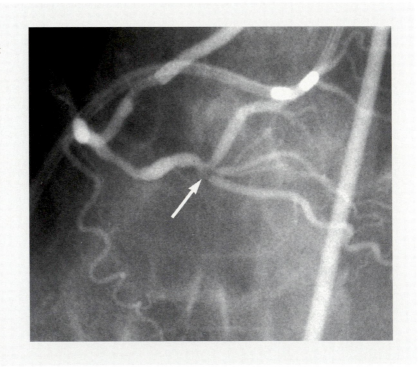

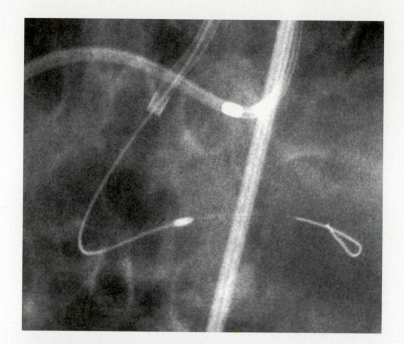

Figure 6.6 B&C
continued

B) A slow pass with a 1.5 mm burr resulted in a perforation due to unfavorable guidewire bias. On severely angulated lesions, pecking or chipping at the lesion is safer since it reduces the amount of time that pressure is placed radially on the arterial wall. Note also the loop in the guidewire in a small distal vessel, which is poor technique. Such angulated, eccentric bifurcation lesions should be treated with extreme caution with the Rotablator system.

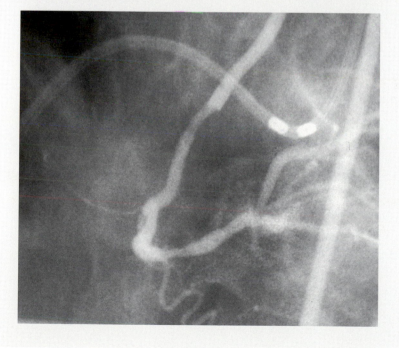

C) A small perforation was treated successfully with PTCA.

Figure 6.7 A-C

Predilation of Side Branch Prior to Rotational Atherectomy

Case Information:
- Guide Catheter: 9 Fr JL-4
- Guidewire: Type C, HI-Torque Floppy
- Pacemaker: No
- Burrs: 1.75, 2.15 mm
- PTCA: 3.0 x 20 mm @ 4 atm.; 2.5 x 20 mm @ 4 atm.

A) This 52 year-old male presented with progressive exertional angina and a complex lesion (arrow) of the LAD and diagonal arteries (Type D). The Type C wire was passed into the LAD and a HI-Torque Floppy into the diagonal. The diagonal was dilated at 4 atm and the balloon and guidewire were removed.

B) The LAD was then treated with 1.75 and 2.15 mm burrs. The 1.75 mm burr was used to treat the more distal LAD lesion as well.

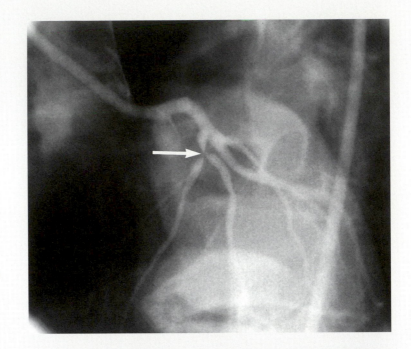

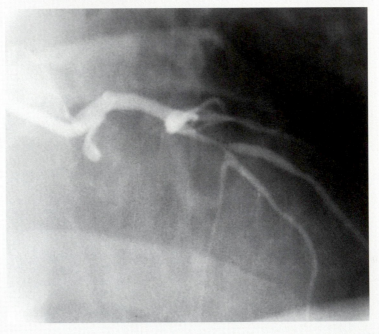

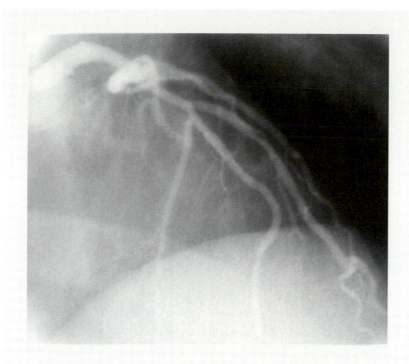

Figure 6.7 C
continued

C) A second Type C wire was placed in the diagonal and the LAD was treated with a 3.0 mm balloon at 4 atm. The wire was removed from the LAD and the diagonal was treated with the 1.75 mm burr. The procedure was completed with "kissing" balloons at 2 atm.

following guidelines when developing a treatment strategy:

- Initiate rotational atherectomy or predilation in the limb in which it is technically more difficult to place the guidewire assuming it is as large, or nearly as large, as the parent vessel.
- Predilation prior to rotational atherectomy may be performed for secondary branch "preservation".
- For adjunctive PTCA generally place a protecting guidewire.
- Post-rotational atherectomy of the parent vessel, vasospasm in the branch vessel should be treated with vasodilators and or low-pressure PTCA.

Bifurcation Lesions Graphic Illustrations and Case Studies

The following case studies provide examples of the treatment of bifurcation lesions.

Figure 6.8 A-F

Bifurcation Lesions

The mainstay of treating bifurcations is branch preservation and achieving adequate lumina in both limbs. The main epicardial vessel can be treated with standard rotational atherectomy techniques. Operators have also taken advantage of directional rotational atherectomy by placing the guidewire into secondary branches that result in different cutting vectors, allowing smaller burrs to achieve large lumens.

Preservation of small diseased vessels (D and F) that branch off the main epicardial vessels can be achieved by: predilating the side branch prior to rotational atherectomy of the main branch and then subsequently performing rotational atherectomy of the side branch if the result was suboptimal. Initially treating the smaller branch with rotational atherectomy is acceptable as long as a guidewire can easily be placed into the main epicardial vessel if spasm occurred.

As discussed, branch ostial disease with severe angulation should be approached with low burr-to-artery ratios followed by adjunctive PTCA.

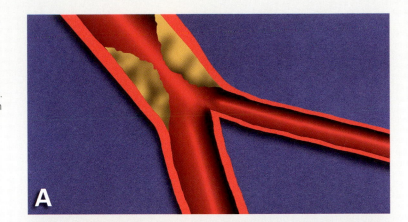

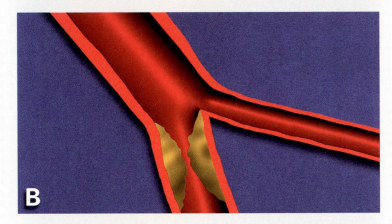

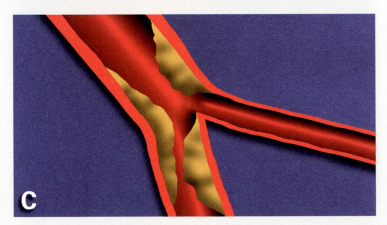

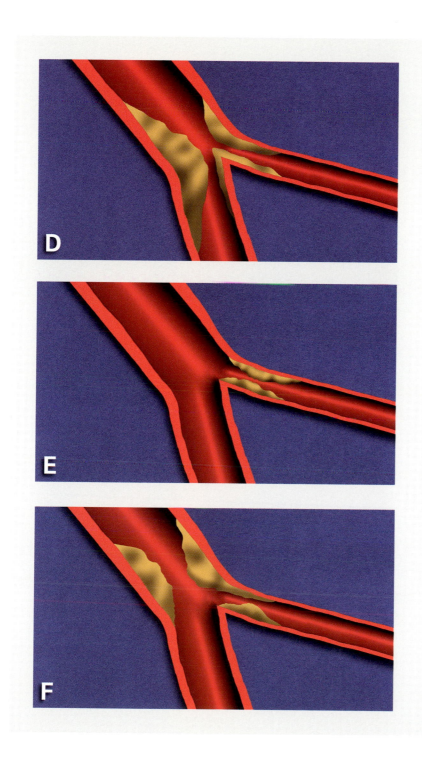

Figure 6.9 A-D

Complex LAD–Diagonal Bifurcation Lesion

Case Information:
- Guide Catheter: JL-3.5
- Guidewire: Type C, HI-Torque Floppy
- Pacemaker: No
- Burrs: 1.5, 2.0 mm
- PTCA: 3.0 x 20 mm; 3.0 x 20 mm

A) This 54 year-old woman with prolonged chest pain and anterior ECG changes had a bifurcation lesion (arrow) with 95% stenosis of the LAD with involvement of the diagonal artery (Type C).

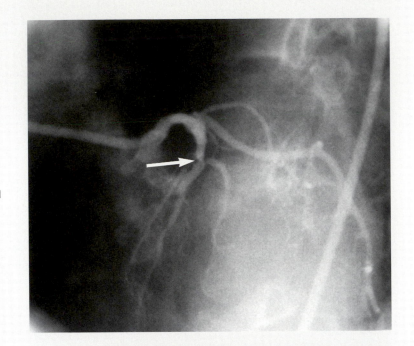

B) The severity of the lesion is more apparent in this RAO cranial projection. The lesion was crossed with a Type C wire placed in the LAD and treated with 1.5 and 2.0 mm burrs. After the 2.0 mm burr there was minimal reduction of flow in the diagonal.

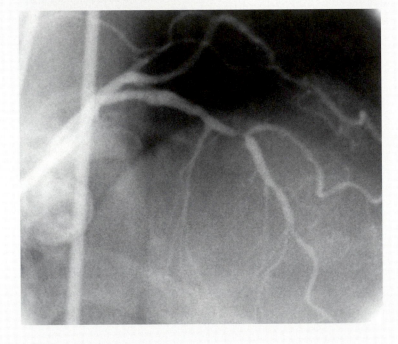

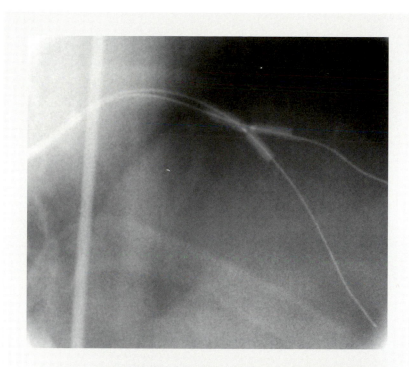

Figure 6.9 C&D
continued

C) Choice™ Floppy guidewires were then passed into the LAD and the diagonal and the vessels were dilated with "kissing" balloons.

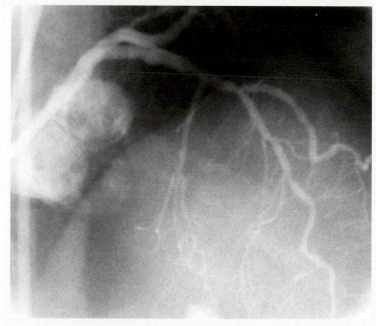

D) Post-treatment there was minimal residual stenosis and TIMI III flow in both branches.

Figure 6.10 A-F

Subtotal Occlusion of Ostial Circumflex and Obtuse Marginal Bifurcation

Case Information:
- Guide Catheter: 8 Fr Voda 3.5
- Guidewire: RotaWire Support
- Pacemaker: No
- Burrs: 1.25 mm
- PTCA: 2.5 x 20 mm @ 6 atm

A) This 64 year-old male continued to suffer angina despite maximal medical therapy. He had a subtotal occlusion at the ostial circumflex (arrow) and lesions in both anterior and posterior limbs of the bifurcation of the circumflex. The 90° angle of the origin of the circumflex limited the burr size which could be safely deployed.

B) The guidewire was placed into the posterior limb which was treated with a 1.25 mm burr.

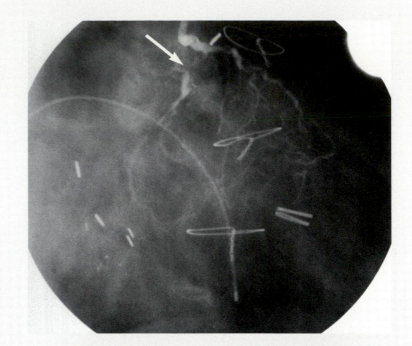

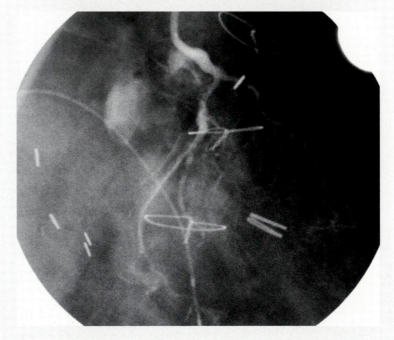

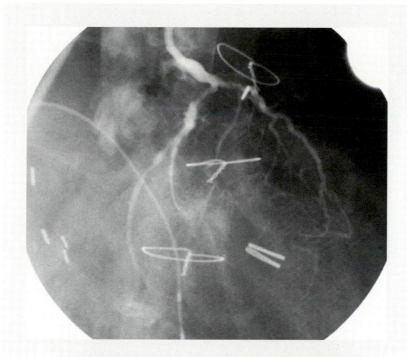

Figure 6.10 C&D
continued

C) The guidewire was then placed into the anterior limb and ablation was repeated with a 1.25 mm burr.

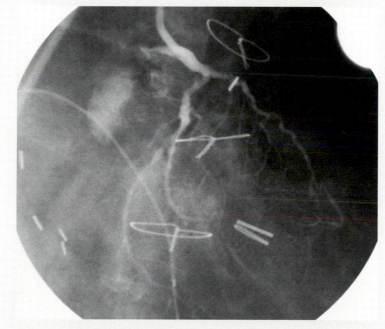

D) Adjunctive PTCA was performed with a 2.5 mm balloon at 6 atm (lesion modification). Larger burrs were not used due to the angulation of the ostial circumflex.

Figure 6.10 E&F
continued

E) Balloon dilation was performed in both limbs as well as in the ostium and proximal circumflex with a 2.5 mm balloon at 6 atm.

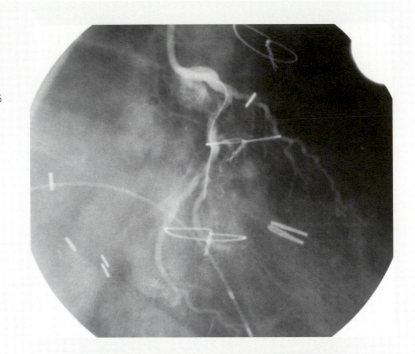

F) The final result demonstrates a 30% residual stenosis of the ostial circumflex and 20% at the bifurcation of the circumflex obtuse marginal.

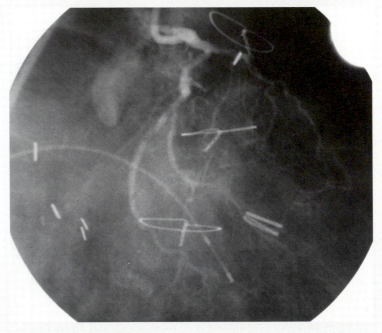

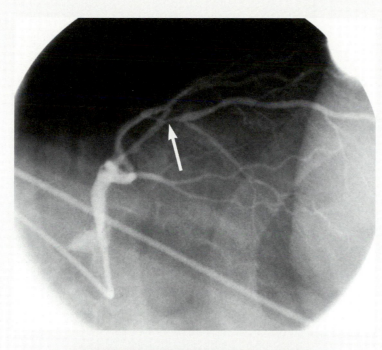

Figure 6.11 A&B

LAD Diagonal Bifurcation

Case Information:
- Guide Catheter: 9 Fr JL-4
- Guidewire: RotaWire Floppy
- Pacemaker: Yes
- Burrs: 1.75, 2.15, 2.25 mm
- PTCA: 3.5 x 20 mm @ 3 atm

A) This 53 year-old male had a mid-LAD lesion at the takeoff of the diagonal (arrow). After crossing the lesion with a RotaWire Floppy, it was treated with 1.75, 2.15 and 2.25 mm burrs.

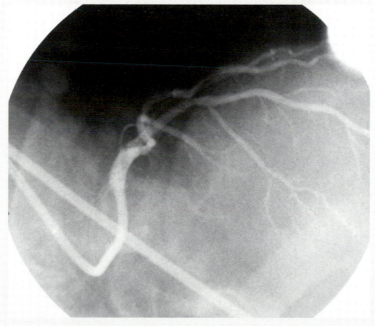

B) Following atherectomy the site was post-dilated with a 3.5 mm balloon at 1 atm. The diagonal remained unperturbed during the procedure.

Figure 6.12 A&B

Circumflex Obtuse Marginal Bifurcation

Case Information:
- Guide Catheter: 8 Fr AL-2
- Guidewire: Type C
- Pacemaker: No
- Burrs: 1.5, 1.75 mm
- PTCA: 2.5 x 20 mm in each limb @ 4 atm

A) This complex lesion (arrow) was treated by lesion modification. The main circumflex and obtuse marginal were each treated with 1.5 and 1.75 mm burrs. In this case the anterior limb which was more difficult to cross was treated first.

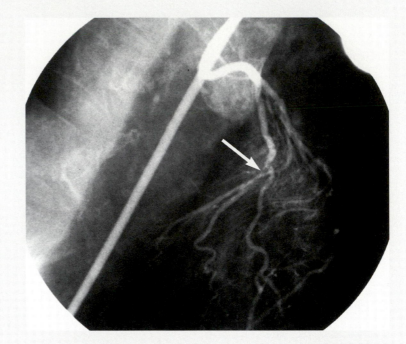

B) After atherectomy of both limbs, balloon dilation was performed with a 2.5 mm balloon.

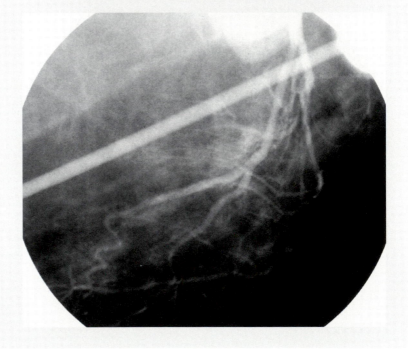

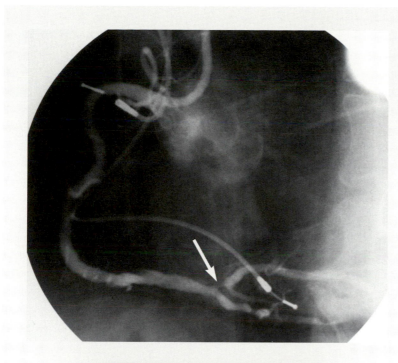

Figure 6.13 A&B

Treatment of Distal Bifurcation

Case Information:
- Guide Catheter: 9 Fr Hockeystick 2
- Guidewire: RotaWire Floppy
- Pacemaker: Yes
- Burrs: 1.75, 2.15 mm
- PTCA: 3.5 x 20 mm @ 1 atm

A) This 46 year-old male returned with restenosis of a distal branch ostial RCA lesion (arrow) which had been treated with rotational atherectomy five months prior with 1.5 and 2.0 mm burrs. The lesion was a focal lesion at the origin of the PDA (Type B).

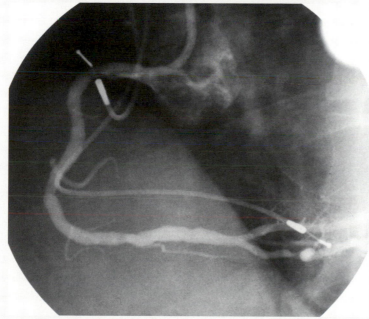

B) Atherectomy was performed with 1.75 and 2.15 mm burrs, slightly larger than used in the original procedure, and was followed by a 3.5 mm balloon at 1 atm. Frequently in restenotic lesions the burrs selected are larger than those used in the first procedure.

Calcified Lesions

Rotational atherectomy has been shown to treat calcified lesions with procedural success equivalent to non-calcified lesions[37] and with procedural success superior to balloon angioplasty.[36] PTCA failures due to inability to dilate or cross the lesion are often calcified and can be successfully managed with rotational atherectomy.[45,46]

The safety and efficacy of the device in these complex lesions has led some catheterization labs to reserve rotational atherectomy for these cases or lesions. Severely calcified lesions have become the "signature lesion" of the Rotablator system.

Guide Catheter:

- Select a guide catheter (with sideholes) that is large enough to accommodate the largest anticipated burr.
- Guide catheters with firm support may be needed in rigid vessels to advance the guidewire and burr to the lesion site.

Guidewire:

- Type C guidewires cross most lesions, provided the vessel is not extremely rigid. In rigid vessels with even minimal tortuosity, the stiff Rotablator Type C guidewire is difficult to advance to distal lesions and conventional guidewire systems may be required first and then exchanged. The RotaWire Floppy appears to be easier to manipulate in these vessels.
- In tortuous rigid vessels, the Rotablator guidewire lies eccentrically in the vessels and can be forced preferentially against the vessel wall (see Figure 3.9). When a guidewire lies eccentrically in the vessel it can become difficult to advance a nonactivated burr. If the burr is activated in these segments the result may be a guttering effect on the vessel. This guttering effect can be seen angiographically as a enlargement of the outer margin of the vessel. Low-speed advancement is suggested if activation of the device is necessary (see Chapter 3 "Burr Advancement Techniques", page 82).

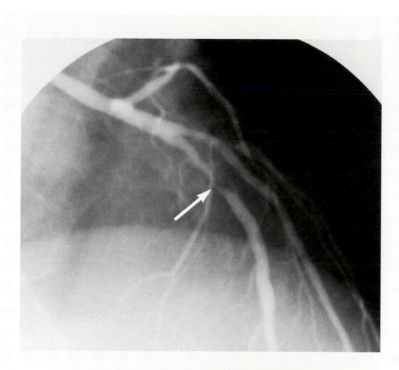

Figure 6.14 A&B

Calcified LAD

Case Information:
- Guide Catheter: 9 Fr JL-4
- Guidewire: Type C
- Pacemaker: No
- Burrs: 1.75, 2.25 mm
- PTCA: 3.5 x 20 mm
  perfusion @ 1atm

A) This heavily calcified mid-LAD lesion (arrow) in a 51 year-old male was treated with primary therapy.

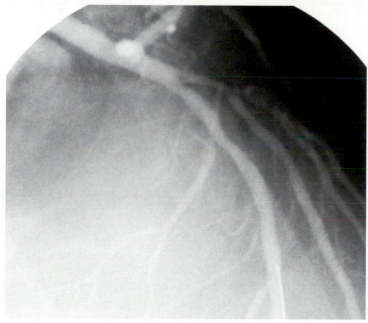

B) After 1.75 and 2.25 mm burrs and a 10 minute 1 atm inflation with a perfusion balloon, there was minimal residual stenosis.

Burr Selection:

- A stepped-burr approach is recommended.
- Undersizing the initial burr is necessary in lesions with moderate to severe calcium. The reasons to undersize the burr include:
  1) Reduction of plaque burden to the distal bed.
  2) Assessment of the clinical response of the patient.
- In heavily calcified lesions, unexpectedly large lumens can be achieved as though the vessel becomes unconstrained as the calcium is removed, or from favorable guidewire bias in an inelastic vessel.
- Interpolated angioplasty is helpful in these lesions. When slow flow occurs PTCA often improves flow and permits use of larger burrs safely.

Ablation Technique:

- Use gentle advancement avoiding decelerations greater than 5,000 rpm, and limiting ablation times to approximately 15 seconds per run. Maintaining short run times and segmental ablation is essential in these lesions.
- During the ablation, contrast injections should be used to assess the orientation of cutting.
- Contrast injections will indicate the flow during the ablation. Frequent burr retractions are essential in order to restore antegrade flow to increase particle clearance.
- The interval between ablation runs should be long enough for the patient's hemodynamics to stabilize and for evidence of unimpaired distal flow.

Strategy:

- Attempt primary therapy with rotational atherectomy. Adjunctive PTCA is minimally effective in highly calcified lesions.
- Any compromises in flow should be corrected prior to use of larger burrs. If the flow is compromised, wait several minutes and, if necessary, perform low-pressure PTCA.
- Larger burrs may be used after PTCA if there is no dissection

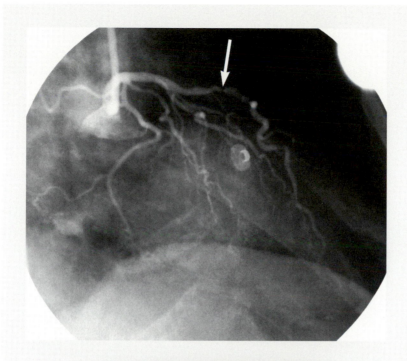

Figure 6.15 A&B
Failed PTCA

Case Information:
- Guide Catheter: 8 Fr JL-4
- Guidewire: RotaWire Support
- Pacemaker: No
- Burr: 1.5 mm
- PTCA: 2.5 x 20 mm @ 4 atm

A) This 73 year-old man had a heavily calcified LAD lesion (arrow). The lesion was difficult to cross and an attempted PTCA at 8 atm was unsuccessful.

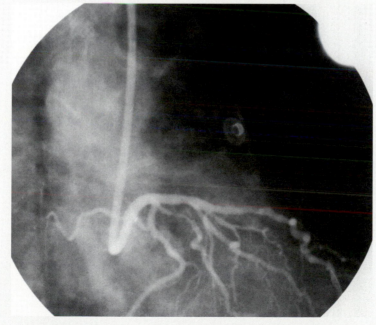

B) The wire was exchanged for a RotaWire Support guidewire. The lesion was treated with a 1.5 mm burr followed by a 2.0 mm balloon at 4 atm with full expansion.

noted angiographically.

- Significant chest discomfort with ECG changes should be corrected prior to use of larger burrs. This situation usually improves by waiting and maintaining adequate hemodynamics.
- If persistent chest pain, ECG changes or flow compromises occur, do not perform further ablation.
- The use of larger burrs may be limited by proximal tortuosity or vessel rigidity.
- If rotastent is the strategy, assess lesion compliance by using PTCA and verify that the balloon fully inflates at 6–7 atm to guarantee full expansion of the stent. If not, use larger burrs prior to stenting to further improve the compliance and reduce plaque mass.

Calcified Lesion Case Studies

These case studies illustrate issues related to calcified lesions.

Figure 6.16 A-E

Interpolated Angioplasty of a Calcified RCA

Case Information:
- Guide Catheter: JR-4
- Guidewire: Type C
- Pacemaker: Yes
- Burr: 1.5, 1.75, 2.0 mm
- PTCA 3.0, @ 1 atm.

A) This heavily calcified mid-RCA lesion (shown in an LAO view) was treated with multiple burrs.

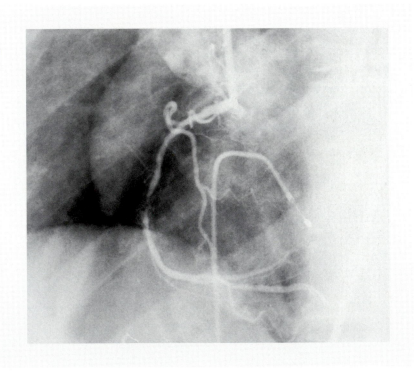

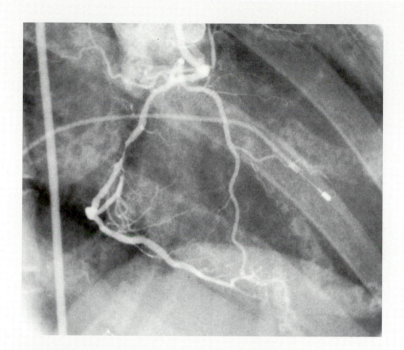

Figure 6.16 B&C
continued

B) The RAO view of the lesion reveals no unsuspected tortuosity which would preclude the use of larger burrs.

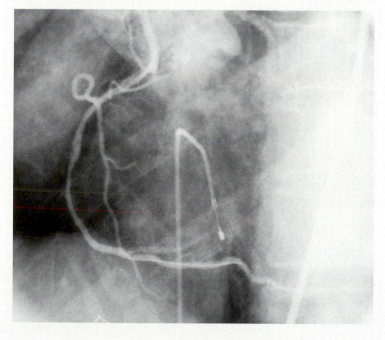

C) After the 1.5 mm burr, PTCA with a 3.0 mm balloon at 1 atm was performed to relieve vasospasm and poor distal flow.

Figure 6.16 D&E
continued

D) Following PTCA the lesion was treated with a 1.75 mm burr, which was complicated by chest pain and vasospasm at the lesion site. The vasospasm was treated with a 3.0 mm balloon at 2 atm.

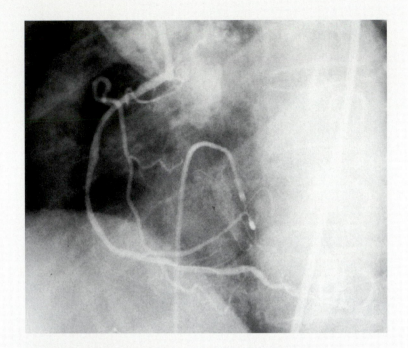

E) The lesion was then ablated with a 2.0 mm burr followed by low-pressure PTCA for this final result.

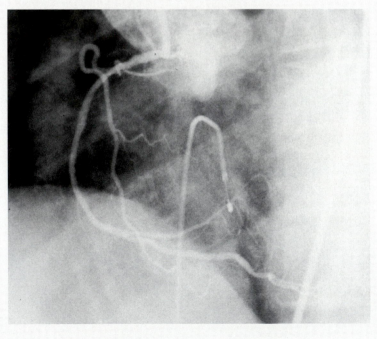

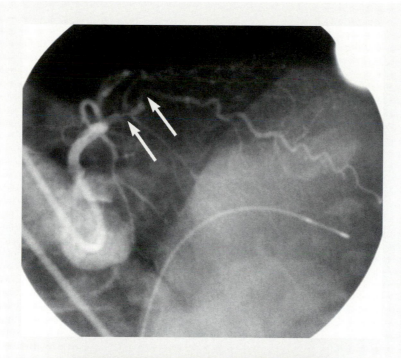

Figure 6.17 A&B

Failed PTCA

Case Information:
- Guide Catheter: AL-1
- Guidewire: Wisdom™,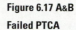
  Type C
- Pacemaker: Yes
- Burrs: 1.5, 2.0 mm
- PTCA: 3.0 x 30 mm
  @ 2 atm

A) After successful rotational atherectomy and stent placement in the RCA, attempts to dilate these mid-LAD lesions (arrows) at 6 atm were unsuccessful. The lesions were subsequently treated with 1.5 and 2.0 mm burrs. (See "Rotational Atherectomy Following Primary PTCA", page 104.)

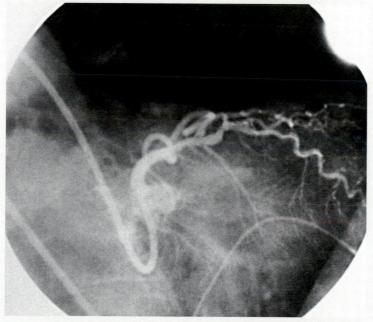

B) The lesions were then easily dilated with a 3.0 mm balloon at 2 atm, confirming an increase in vessel compliance. Due to heavy calcification and the treatment of multiple arteries, ReoPro was used during the procedure.

Figure 6.18 A-D

**Guidewire Bias in
Rigid Vessel**

Case Information:
- Guide Catheter: 9 Fr
  Hockeystick
- Guidewire: Type C
- Pacemaker: Yes
- Burrs: 1.5, 2.0 and
  2.25 mm
- PTCA: 3.5 x 20 mm
  @ 4 atm

A) This heavily calcified RCA
in an 89 year-old female,
has lesions in the mid and
distal RCA.

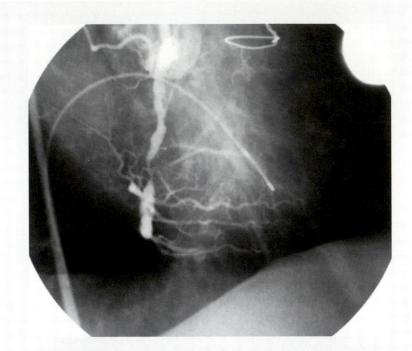

B) The RAO view
demonstrates a moderately
stenosed segment (arrow)
proximal to the lesion.

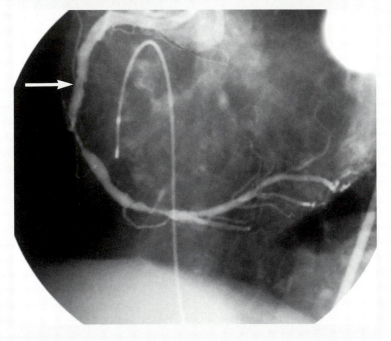

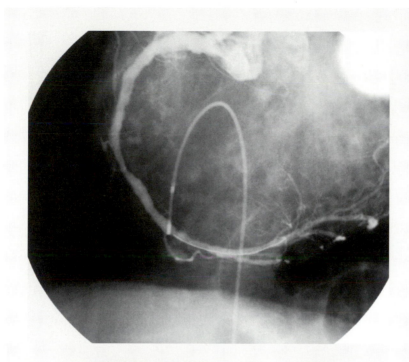

Figure 6.18 C&D
continued

C) The mid and distal lesions were treated with 1.5 and 2.0 mm burrs. Despite multiple attempts at gentle advancement, a 2.25 mm burr would not cross the lesion due to the guidewire bias which caused the burr to vector tangentially.

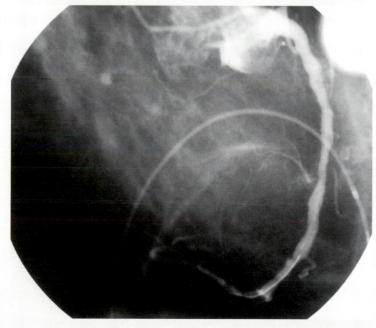

D) Treatment was completed with a 3.5 mm balloon at 4 atm. The final result is shown in the left lateral view.

Eccentric Lesions

Debulking in eccentric lesions requires attention to all the nuances of proper technique. The guidewire plays an important role in the efficiency of debulking these lesions. In addition, very slow passes are recommended to ensure the burr doesn't "slip" or "watermelon seed" across the lesion. After each burr treatment, conduct a critical analysis of the lumen achieved.

Guide Catheter:
- Select a guide catheter (with sideholes) that is large enough to accommodate the largest anticipated burr.
- Assess possible positions of the guide catheter and the impact on the guidewire. (Refer to Chapter 3 "Guidewire Positioning and Guidewire Bias", page 52.)
- Use active guidewire technique by manipulating the guide catheter to orient guidewire towards the lesion if necessary.

Guidewire:
- Standard guidewire techniques should be followed.
- May be able to direct guidewire over the lesion (preferential ablation) for directional rotational atherectomy. (Figure 3.15, page 66).
- A Type C or RotaWire Extra Support guidewire may be advantageous over the RotaWire Floppy guidewire since with favorable guidewire bias it can place more tension on the lesion because of its stiffness.

Burr Selection:
- A stepped-burr approach is recommended. Undersize the initial burr (typically by 0.5 mm).
- Smaller incremental burr sizes should be considered to compensate for "directional" debulking that takes place when the burr is ablating preferentially in the lesion.

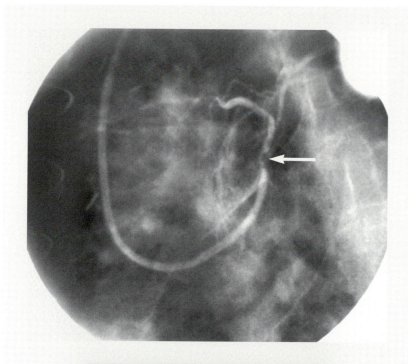

Figure 6.19 A&B

Eccentric Lesion of LAD

Case Information:
- Guide Catheter: 8 Fr JL-4
- Guidewire: Type C
- Pacemaker: No
- Burrs: 1.5 mm
- PTCA: 3.0 x 30 mm
  @ 6 atm

A) This 75 year-old man with a history of two bypass surgeries was admitted for increasing angina. The 95% eccentric stenosis in the LAD (arrow) was treated with a 1.5 mm burr. The lumen was larger than anticipated due to favorable guidewire bias directing the burr into the eccentric lesion. The procedure was completed with angioplasty.

B) Post-balloon, the lesion was well dilated with notably better flow into a very large first septal.

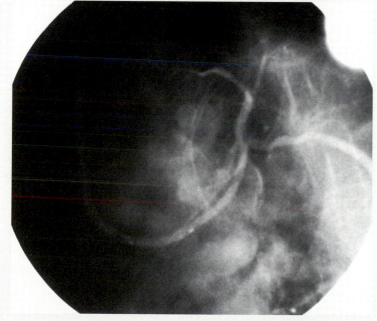

Ablation Technique:

- Use gentle advancement avoiding decelerations greater than 5,000 rpm and keep ablation time to 15–30 sec./run.
- Use contrast injections to assess the relation of the burr to the lesion.
- Advance the burr slowly and make several "polishing" runs to thoroughly treat the lesion; otherwise, if the burr is advanced too quickly, the burr may "slip" past or "watermelon seed" through the diseased eccentric segment .
- Consider redirecting the guide catheter or "pulling" on the guidewire during ablation to increase the "purchase" on the lesion.

Strategy:

- After initially ablating with a small device, it may be evident that the burr is being oriented to the lesion and "directional ablation" is occurring. In this instance, either make smaller burr size increases or if the lesion is adequately debulked proceed with adjunctive therapy.
- The guidewire may direct the burr away from the lesion and cause the burr to simply glide past the lesion. Ablation of normal tissue in these cases can cause the lumen to appear hazy and may result in dissections if incrementally larger burr sizes are subsequently used.
- A synergy with stents can be performed in large eccentric lesions with the Rotablator system, especially in cases where lesion engagement is difficult due to unfavorable guidewire bias directing the guidewire away from the plaque.

Tortuous Vessels

Tortuosity, when severe, can significantly impact the use of the Rotablator system and make these lesions the most difficult to treat specifically when selecting burr sizes. Guidewire issues are of particular concern (Figure 3.14, page 64).[71]

Guide Catheter

- Select a guide catheter (with sideholes) that is large enough to

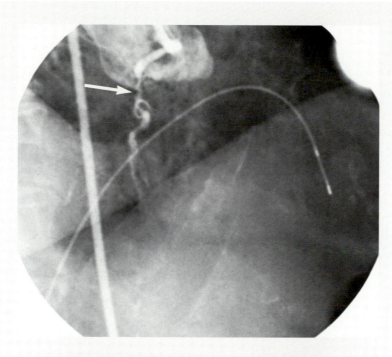

Figure 6.20 A&B

Tortuous RCA

Case Information:
- Guide Catheter: 8 Fr Hockeystick
- Guidewire: RotaWire Floppy
- Pacemaker: Yes
- Burrs: 1.5, 2.0 mm
- PTCA: 3.5 x 30 mm @ 18 atm
- Stent: 1 x PS1530

A) This 80 year-old female had a heavily calcified tortuous lesion in the proximal RCA (arrow). Due to vein stripping she was not a bypass candidate. The lesion was treated with 1.5 and 2.0 mm burrs. Complete inflation of a 3.5 mm balloon at 2 atm indicated that stenting without additional atherectomy was appropriate.

B) A PS1530 stent was implanted and post inflated to 18 atm with this final result. Treatment with rotational atherectomy in the left coronary system followed.

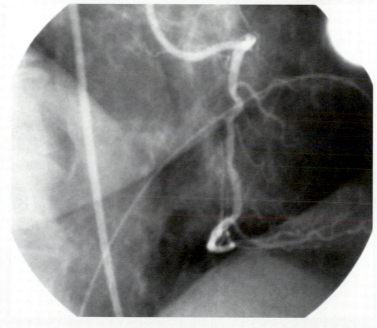

Figure 6.21 A&B

Tortuous RCA

Case Information:
- Guide Catheter: 8 Fr Hockeystick
- Guidewire: HI-Torque Floppy, Type C
- Pacemaker: Yes
- Burrs: 1.25, 1.5 mm
- PTCA: 3.0 x 30 mm @ 2 atm

A) The 90% stenosis of the proximal RCA and the tortuous nature of the vessel distal to the lesion are evident. Note the very proximal placement of the platinum tip of the guidewire (arrow). Because of guidewire bias and the tortuous nature of the vessel, a 1.25 mm burr was used for the initial treatment followed by a 1.5 mm burr. Because of the eccentricity of the lesion and risk of perforation large burrs were not used.

B) Atherectomy was followed by a 3.0 mm balloon dilated to 2 atm with the result shown.

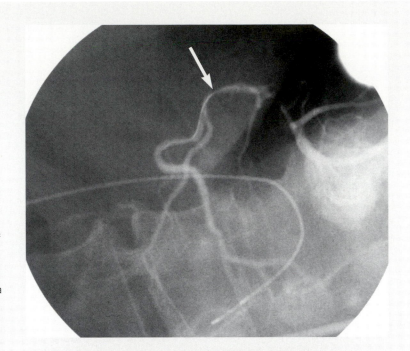

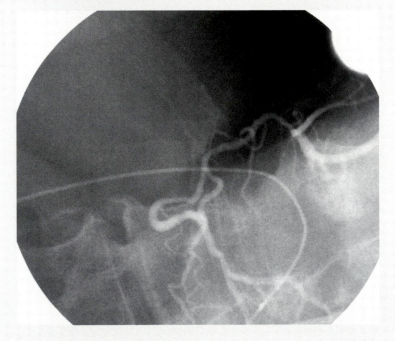

accommodate the largest anticipated burr.

- A guide catheter which is coaxial and with good support is more important in cases with tortuosity.

Guidewire

- In the event of distal tortuosity, the guidewire can cause vessel deformity or "pseudolesions" (see Figure 3.13). In these circumstances retracting the guidewire to as proximal a position as possible will often relieve this problem.
- The RotaWire Floppy guidewire may be advantageous in these lesions.

Burr Selection

- A stepped-burr approach is recommended.
- With proximal tortuosity, the guidewire may deform the vessel making advancement of the nonactivated burr virtually impossible and may limit the maximal burr size.
- Use low-speed advancement technique (100,000 rpm) through these segments. Larger burrs may be difficult to advance and generally should be avoided.
- Proximal tortuosity is often the limiting step for incremental burr sizing.

Ablation Technique

- Use gentle advancement avoiding decelerations greater than 5,000 rpm and keeping ablation times to 15–30 sec./run.
- Activating the burr in segments where the guidewire deforms the vessel is a concern since ablation of normal tissue can occur if the tension on the wall exceeds the elasticity of the vessel.
- Contrast injection during the ablation run is critical to assess how the proximal tortuosity "sets" the cutting vector.

Strategy

- When difficulty is experienced in advancing larger burrs to the lesion, a strategy of lesion modification should be applied.

Restenotic Lesions

Rotational atherectomy has been used frequently in restenotic lesions.[49] By applying a different technology other than PTCA to the lesion, it is hoped that future restenosis will be reduced. This patient subset is ideal for operators to gain familiarity with the device, since these lesions appear to have a lower incidence of vasospasm, slow flow and no reflow.

Guide Catheter:
- Select a guide catheter (with sideholes) that is large enough to accommodate the largest anticipated burr.
- Use conventional shapes in the appropriate sizes.

Guidewire:
- These lesions are usually crossed with a RotaWire Floppy or a Type C guidewire.

Burr Selection:
- A stepped-burr approach is recommended.
- Restenotic lesions are generally treated with two burrs with or without adjunctive low-pressure PTCA. In Rotablator restenotic lesions, the final burr is often 0.25 mm larger than that at of the initial procedure.

Ablation Technique:
- Use gentle advancement avoiding decelerations greater than 5,000 rpm and keeping ablation times to 15–30 sec./run.

Strategy:
- In the absence of randomized clinical trial data, the operator has discretion which strategy to apply in these lesions since high acute procedural success is achievable with almost all the technologies.

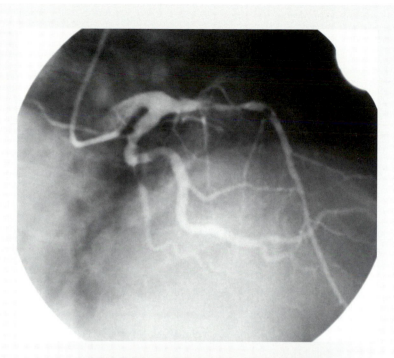

Figure 6.22 A&B

Restenotic Lesions

Case Information:
- Guide Catheter: 9 Fr, JL-4
- Guidewire: Type C
- Pacemaker: No
- Burrs: 1.75, 2.15 mm
- PTCA: 3.0 mm @ 18 atm
- Stent: 2 x PS1530

A) This 67 year-old man had restenosis in the mid-LAD 3 months post-rotational atherectomy which used 1.5 and 2.0 mm burrs.

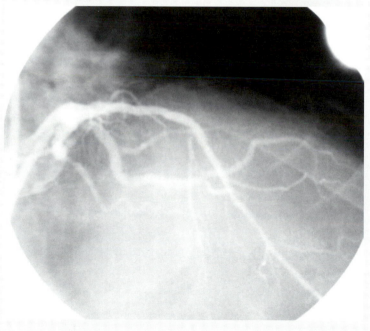

B) The lesion was treated with 1.75 and 2.15 mm burrs followed by two PS1530 stents.

Total Occlusions

Total occlusions, specifically chronic total occlusions which often have fibrocalcific morphologies, are well suited for rotational atherectomy and treatment is limited only by the ability to cross the lesion with the guidewire.[34,72,73,74] Acute occlusions are generally not treated with rotational atherectomy since the substrate is typically thrombus.

Guide Catheter:

- Select a guide catheter (with sideholes) that is large enough to accommodate the largest anticipated burr.
- Standard curves with good support for crossing these frequently difficult lesions may be advantageous.

Guidewire:

- In most cases, the recommendation is to use conventional guidewires and exchange for the Rotablator guidewire with a transfer catheter.
- The Type A guidewire due to its stiffer, shorter tip has similar stiffness to PTCA standard guidewires. However, because the "steerability" of this wire is limited, it is typically reserved for total occlusions in straight segments.

Burr Selection:

- A stepped-burr approach is recommended.
- Initiating treatment with small burrs (1.25 mm) is the safest approach since the position of the guidewire is often not certain when there is no antegrade flow (pilot hole).
- If flow is established by placing the guidewire, treatment should follow standard sizing.
- Once the guidewire is confirmed to be intraluminal, burrs can be increased incrementally.

Ablation Technique:

- Use gentle advancement avoiding decelerations greater than

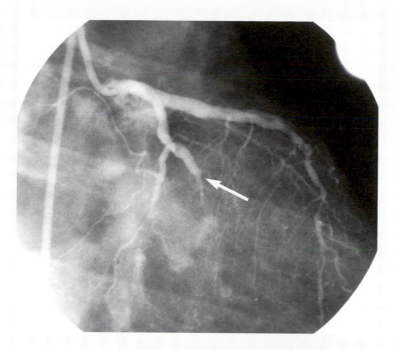

Figure 6.23 A&B

Chronic Total Occlusion

Case Information:
- Guide Catheter: 9 Fr AL-2
- Guidewire: Type C
- Pacemaker: No
- Burrs: 1.5 mm
- PTCA: 3.0 x 20 mm @ 4 atm

A) This total occlusion of the obtuse marginal branch (arrow) was crossed with a Choice Floppy guidewire which was exchanged for a Type C wire. After placement of the wire, antegrade flow was observed and treatment was initiated with a 1.5 mm burr. In the absence of flow, a smaller burr would have been selected.

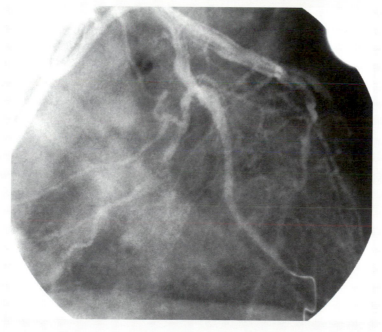

B) Rotational atherectomy was followed by balloon angioplasty. Note that in this case the guidewire is in a small branch. Optimally, it should have been placed more proximally.

5,000 rpm and keeping ablation times 15–30 sec./run.

- In this lesion subset, specifically in cases where the true lumen is not identified, use small burrs and gentle advancement.
- If the burr speed decelerates abruptly (more than 10,000 rpm) this can signal the potential intramural position of the guidewire. The burr should be immediately withdrawn and contrast injected to assess whether vessel trauma has occurred.
- Despite the absence of distal runoff, slow flow has not been identified with an increased frequency in this lesion subset.

Strategy:

- Initiate the procedure with small devices. In total occlusions competitive flow may limit antegrade flow after the initial burr. PTCA at this point can be helpful to ascertain guidewire placement and distal flow. Subsequent burrs can then be used.
- In these complicated lesions, small increases in burr size (0.25 mm) may be necessary since significant distal tapering may not be fully appreciated.
- Interpolated angioplasty (see Chapter 3, "Interpolated Angioplasty", page 106) can improve flow and visualization of the distal vessel, especially in cases with competitive retrograde flow from collaterals.

Total Occlusion Case Studies

The following three case studies illustrate the of treatment chronic total occlusions. Common issues are the ability to cross the lesion with the guidewire and burr sizing. Utilization of small burrs and small burr increments to avoid oversized burrs is warranted until a pilot channel is established and the size of the distal vessel is known. Competitive flow from collaterals and vasospasm may occur more frequently but slow flow has not been seen with increased frequency. It should be reemphasized chronic and not acute (thrombus laden) total occlusions are selected for rotational atherectomy.

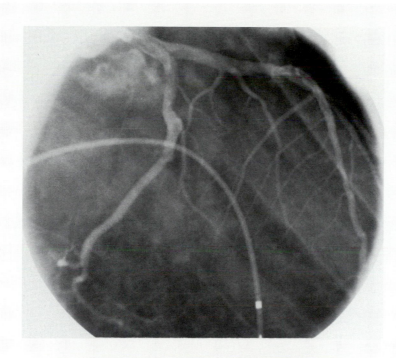

Figure 6.24 A&B

Total Occlusion of an Obtuse Marginal

Case Information:
- Guide Catheter: 9 Fr AL2
- Guidewire: Type C
- Pacemaker: Yes
- Burrs: 1.25, 1.5, 2.0 mm
- PTCA: 3.0 x 20 mm
  @ 4 atm.

A) This chronic total occlusion of an obtuse marginal was crossed with a conventional PTCA guidewire. After exchange for a Type C guidewire, treatment was initiated with a 1.25 mm burr.

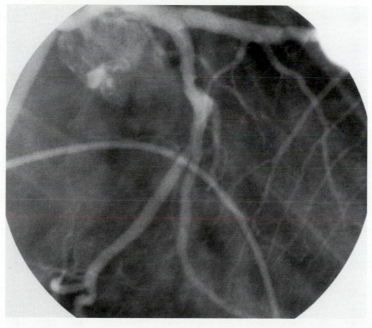

B) After the pilot channel was established, a small burr increment (1.25 to 1.5 mm) was used since the size of the distal vessel was uncertain. With the size of the distal vessel apparent, the 1.5 mm burr was followed by a 2.0 mm burr. PTCA was performed with a 3.0 mm balloon at 4 atm.

Figure 6.25 A-H

Total Occlusion of the LAD

Case Information:
- Guide Catheter: 9 Fr JL-4
- Guidewire: ACS intermediate wire exchanged for Type C
- Pacemaker: No
- Burrs: 1.5, 2.0 mm
- PTCA: 3.5 x 20 mm @ 2 atm

A) This 49 year-old male experienced exertional angina at low work loads and was found to have a subtotal occlusion of the LAD.

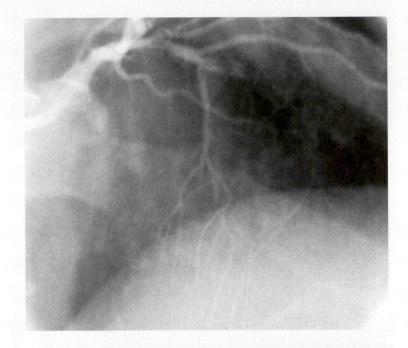

B) An intermediate guidewire was used to cross the lesion. With guidewire placement, antegrade flow (arrow) was visible.

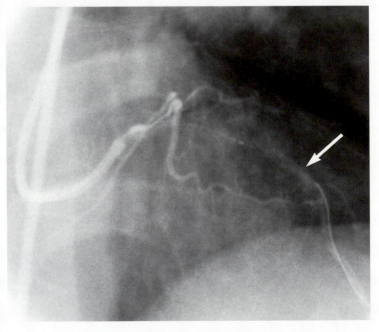

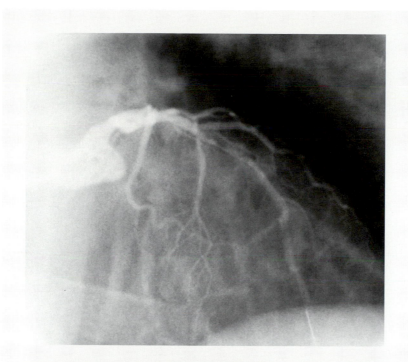

Figure 6.25 C&D
continued

C) Since heavy calcification prohibited a transfer catheter from crossing, the intermediate wire was removed, and a Type C guidewire was successfully placed. The length of the occlusion was 15 mm with a moderate size distal vessel.

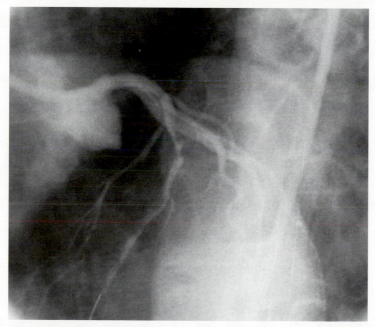

D) This LAO projection shows the lesion with the distal vessel beyond.

Figure 6.25 E&F
continued

E) Because flow had been established and the distal vessel size was known, treatment was initiated with a 1.5 mm burr.

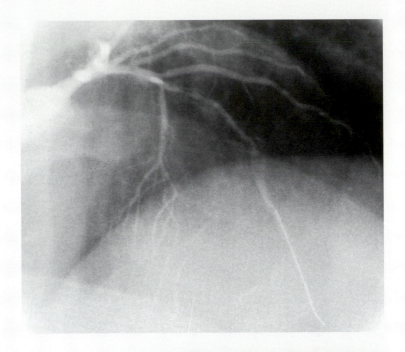

F) After the 1.5 mm burr the channel is open and flow is improved in the distal vessel.

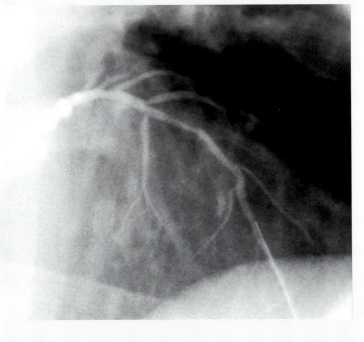

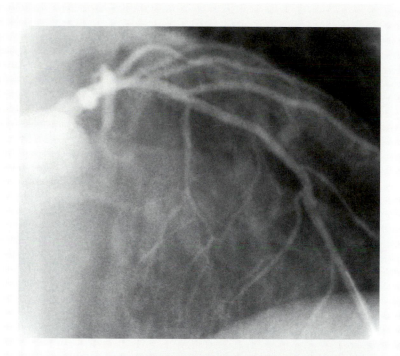

Figure 6.25 G&H
continued

G) After upsizing to a 2.0 mm burr there was a good angiographic result with normal antegrade flow.

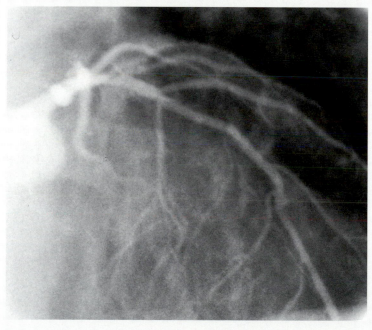

H) Low-pressure balloon inflation post-atherectomy was performed with a 3.5 mm balloon yielding this final result.

Figure 6.26 A-D

Total Occlusion of LAD with Platforming in Left Main

Case Information:
- Guide Catheter: 8 Fr JL-4
- Guidewire: Type C
- Pacemaker: Yes
- Burrs: 1.25, 1.5, 1.75 and 2.0 mm
- PTCA: 3.5 x 4.0 mm @ 1 atm

A) This total occlusion (arrow) of the LAD in a 48 year-old university professor without previous MI was treated with primary therapy using multiple burrs. The vessel was diffusely diseased and required ablation from the ostium to the distal LAD. Platforming in the left main was required.

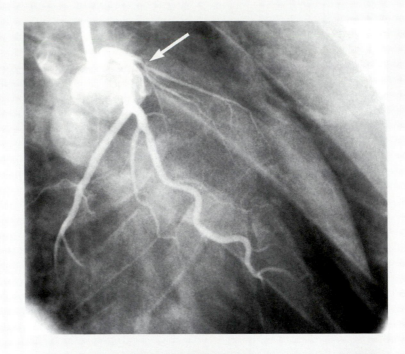

B) Because there was minimal flow after placement of the guidewire, vessel diameter could not be determined, and treatment was initiated with a 1.25 mm burr.

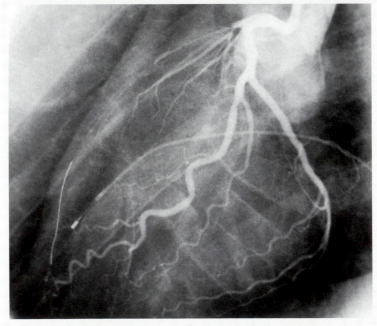

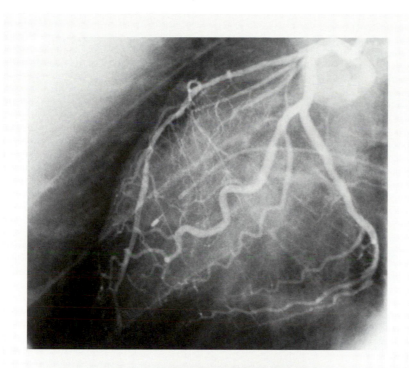

Figure 6.26 C&D
continued

C) Treatment with the
1.25 mm burr was followed
with 1.5 and 1.75 mm burrs.
Intravascular ultrasound
revealed significant residual
disease with an estimated
vessel size of 3.5 to 4.0 mm.
Atherectomy with a 2.0 mm
burr was performed followed
by a 3.5 x 40 mm balloon at
1 atm using several inflations
along the length of the vessel.

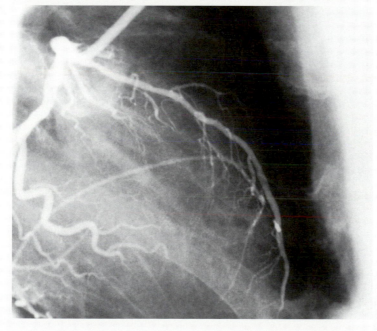

D) Final angiogram from RAO
projection reveals a 10%
residual stenosis with good
antegrade flow.

Long Lesions

Long lesions are defined as lesions greater than 15 mm in length. The potential for large quantities of plaque generated in these cases, has led to several technique modifications to reduce adverse outcomes such as slow and no reflow. Challenges in treating this lesion subset include guidewire placement and appropriate burr sizing sequence to minimize the plaque burden.[30, 39]

Guide Catheter:

- Select a guide catheter (with sideholes) that is large enough to accommodate the largest anticipated burr and provides adequate support. The Rotablator guidewire will often lose a great deal of pushability as it negotiates diffusely diseased segments. Good backup from the guide catheter can be helpful.

Guidewire:

- If a long lesion is significantly complex, use conventional angioplasty wires and exchange through low-profile balloons or transfer catheters. In most cases, the more flexible tip on the Type C guidewire should be used. However, if the lesion is very distal and there is limited vessel length beyond the lesion, the Type A can be used. The new generation RotaWire guidewires may prove superior in tracking to the Type C or A guidewires in these lesions.

Burr Selection:

- A stepped-burr approach is recommended.
- Burr selection is determined by the anticipated plaque burden, the ratio of lesion length to distal runoff, and the ventricular function in the territory subtended by the vessel. These cases commonly require two burrs, and in some cases, three.
- If larger burrs are used, contrast injections during the ablation will help confirm that an oversized burr is not advanced into a small distal segment.
- Small incremental steps (i.e. 0.25 mm) will minimize plaque

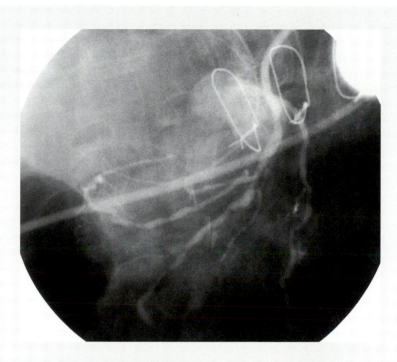

Figure 6.27 A&B

Long Lesion of Circumflex

Case Information:
- Guide Catheter: 8 Fr Voda 3.5
- Guidewire: RotaWire Support
- Pacemaker: Yes
- Burrs: 1.5, 1.75 mm
- PTCA: 3.0 x 30 mm @ 4 atm.

A) This 78 year-old woman presented with increasing angina and this long diffuse lesion of the circumflex with a mid-segment bridging ectasia.

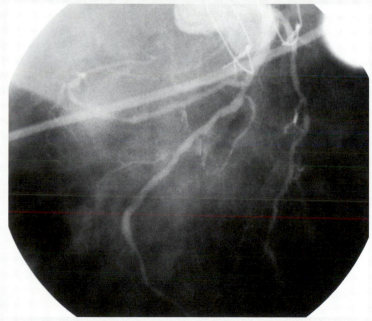

B) The lesion was treated with 1.5 and 1.75 mm burrs followed by a 3.0 mm long balloon at 4 atm for this final result.

burden and is suggested in extremely long lesions.

- Interpolated angioplasty can be helpful in these cases. (See Chapter 3, "Interpolated Angioplasty", page 106.)

Ablation Technique:

- Use gentle advancement avoiding decelerations greater than 5,000 rpm and keeping ablation times to 15–30 sec./run.
- The lesion should be treated with segmental ablation. The total lesion need not be ablated during a single run.
- Time should be taken between ablations to permit the clearance of particles and the administration of vasodilators if necessary.
- Between ablation runs, the burr should be positioned such that it does not limit flow.

Strategy:

- Smaller steps in burr sizes are advocated in long lesions especially in cases with other complex features such as calcium.
- If there is significant chest discomfort, ECG changes, or hemodynamic compromise during ablation runs with the initial burr, then larger burrs should not be used until improvement or resolution of clinical or angiographic compromise.
- PTCA, with low-pressure inflations, or subselective nitroglycerin can improve flow between runs prior to a step up in burrs (interpolated angioplasty).
- Long balloons offer excellent adjunctive therapy.
- Adjunctive ReoPro should be considered in these cases since long lesions often require long ablation times.

Long Lesion Case Studies:

Lesions greater than 15 mm in length offer challenges in selecting burr sequences and ablation techniques to minimize the impact of the large plaque burden. Undersizing the initial burr, using segmental ablation and treating with lower pressure angioplasty between burrs (interpolated angioplasty) may help to improve particle clearance.

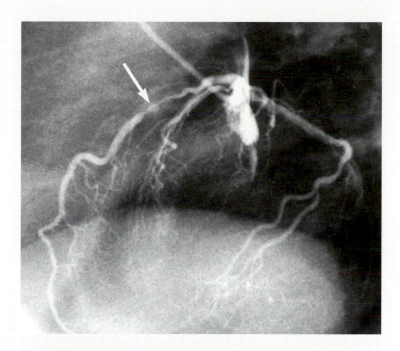

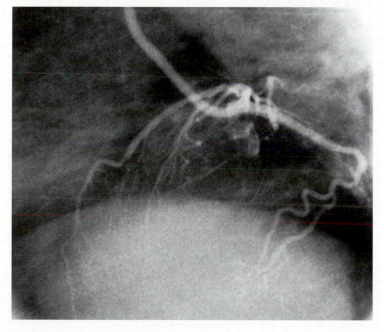

Figure 6.28 A&B

**Segmental Ablation
of the LAD**

Case Information:
- Guide Catheter: JL-4
- Guidewire: Type C
- Pacemaker: No
- Burrs: 1.5, 2.0 mm
- PTCA: 3.0 x 40 mm,
  @ 1 atm

A) This 40 mm long LAD
lesion (arrow) was treated
with segmental ablation
(15–30 seconds). It required
six separate runs to
completely treat the lesion.

B) Post-treatment there was
a 20% residual stenosis and
excellent flow.

Figure 6.29 A-D

Long Lesion of RCA

Case Information:
- Guide Catheter: 8 Fr JR-4
- Guidewire: RotaWire Floppy
- Pacemaker: Yes
- Burrs: 1.25, 1.5 mm
- PTCA: 3.0 x 20 mm @ 2 atm

A) This 76 year-old female presented with increasing angina and a long calcified lesion that extended from proximal to mid-RCA.

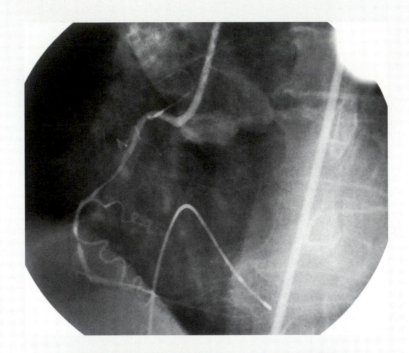

B) After placement of a RotaWire Floppy guidewire, there was only slight distortion of the vessel.

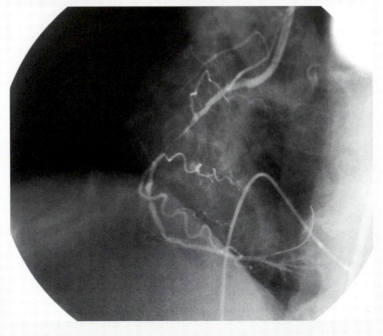

Figure 6.29 C&D
continued

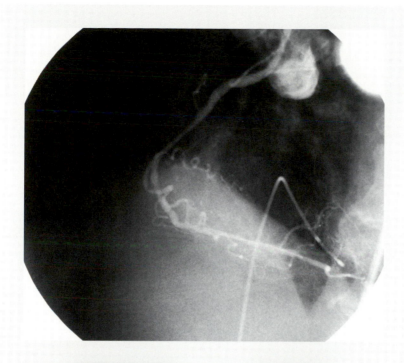

C) The lesion was treated with 1.25 and 1.5 mm burrs, using segmental ablation.

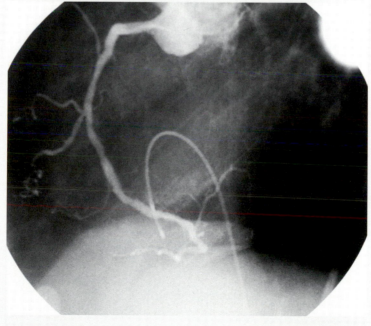

D) After atherectomy the vessel was dilated with a 3.0 mm balloon at low pressure.

Rotastent

Stenting has taken a prominent position in percutaneous revascularization due to improved long-term results when compared to balloon angioplasty, as reported in the Benestent and STRESS trials.[78,79] These trials targeted lesions in larger vessels with minimal complexity. The question becomes: can stenting achieve comparable outcomes in lesions with less favorable characteristics?

To determine the viability of expanded indications for stenting, two strategies can be applied. One strategy is to simply "push the envelope" of stenting, and see whether clinical trials can replicate the success of stents in a less favorable lesion subset. This approach may have little justification considering the difficulty of stent delivery, and optimal deployment in calcified and diffusely diseased vessels.

The second approach, based on the concept of "lesion modification", is to simplify the complexity of the lesion with rotational atherectomy prior to stent deployment. Debulking increases vessel compliance, reduces plaque mass which can ease stent delivery, and allow greater lumen expansion.[57,58,75] Rotational atherectomy generally creates a smooth, round lumen, and provides greater opportunity for concentric stent apposition. The integration of second-generation devices offers new and exciting directions in interventional cardiology.

Guide Catheter:

- Select a guide catheter (with sideholes) that is large enough to accommodate the largest anticipated burr.
- Use conventional shapes.
- The guide catheter selected should be the "optimal" for stenting.
- If visualization for stent deployment is anticipated to be difficult with sidehole catheters, using a larger guide catheter may be helpful.

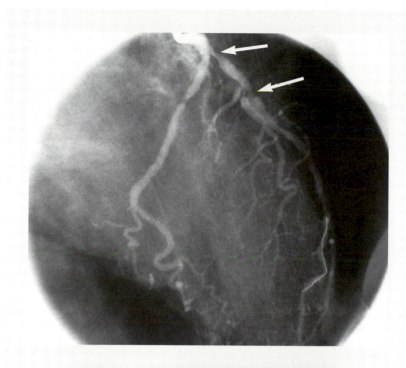

Figure 6.30 A&B

Rotastent of the LAD

Case Information:
- Guide Catheter: 8 Fr JL-4
- Guidewire: Type C for RA, Extra Support for stent
- Pacemaker: No
- Burr: 1.5 mm
- PTCA: 3.5 x 20 mm @ 18 atm.
- Stent: 2 x PS1530

A) These heavily calcified complex proximal LAD lesions (arrows) were treated with a 1.5 mm burr to ease stent deployment and increase vessel compliance.

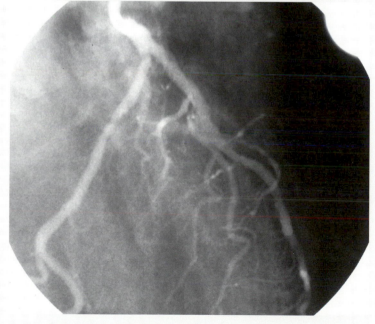

B) This vessel is shown after treatment with a single burr and placement of 2 stents at high pressures.

Figure 6.31 A&B

Rotastent of Subtotal Occlusion of the RCA

Case Information:
- Guide Catheter: 8 Fr JR-4
- Guidewire: Type C
- Pacemaker: Yes
- Burr: 1.5 mm
- PTCA: 3.5 x 20 mm, @ 18 atms.
- Stent: 3 x PS1530

A) The long subtotal occlusion of the RCA was treated with a single undersized burr (1.5 mm) to ease stent deployment and increase vessel compliance.

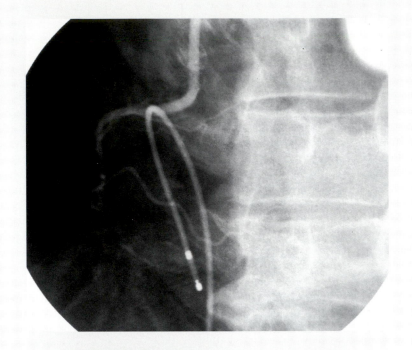

B) There is no residual stenosis after three PS1530 stents.

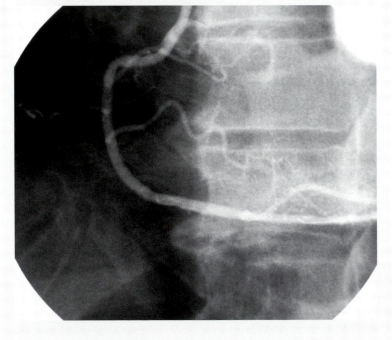

Guidewire:
- Depending on the lesion morphology and vessel characteristics, a RotaWire Floppy or Extra Support guidewire is selected.
- In the majority of cases prior to stenting the Rotablator guidewire is exchanged for a conventional guidewire that would be used for stent deployment.

Burr Selection:
- A stepped-burr approach is recommended.
- Follow guidelines for lesion morphology.

Ablation Technique:
- Use gentle advancement avoiding decelerations greater than 5,000 rpm and keep ablation times to 15–30 sec./run.
- Follow guidelines for lesion morphology.

Strategy:
The optimal strategies are presently being defined. Below are several options:
- Minimal debulking: use a single undersized burr to debulk and modify the vessel compliance. Assess compliance with balloon inflation prior to stent placement to be certain adequate debulking is accomplished to permit expansion. Typically PTCA is performed at 6 atm. If the balloon has a "waist" then further debulking is suggested.
- Maximal debulking: conventional step-procedure followed by placement of the stent (some operators will still predilate, but typically with the final anticipated balloon).
- Balloon pressures: The majority of operators maintain the use of high-pressure PTCA after rotastenting.

Rotastent Graphic Illustrations and Case Studies
The case studies and illustrations which follow demonstrate some of the issues associated with rotastenting.

Figure 6.32 A-D

Stent Deployment

This series shows the conventional deployment of a stent in an artery without prior debulking. Atherosclerotic plaque is displaced by the stent into the surrounding tissue.

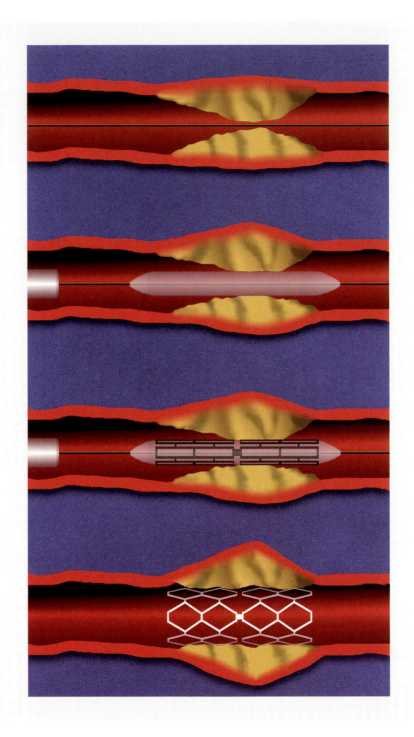

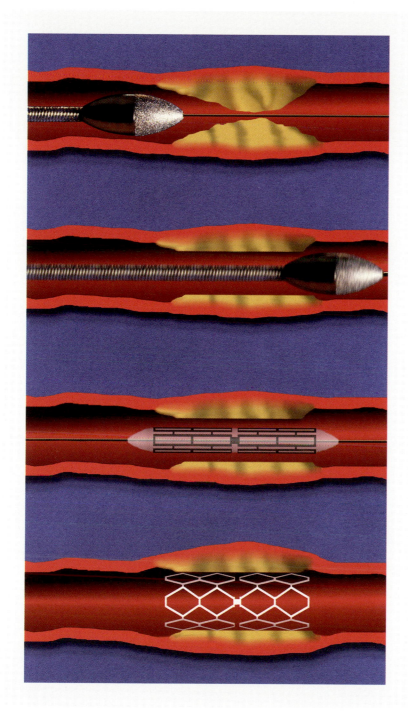

Figure 6.32 E-H

Rotastent Procedure

In this sequence rotational atherectomy is performed to remove atherosclerotic plaque which may be beneficial in improving stent deployment and obtaining more concentric and larger lumens. The decrease in vessel stretch (plaque displacement) post-ablation may also have consequences on long-term outcome. A multicenter trial will compare rotastent vs. PTCA-stent.

Figure 6.33 A-D

Rotastent of the Proximal RCA

Case Information:
- Guide Catheter: 8 Fr Hockeystick
- Guidewire: Type C
- Pacemaker: Yes
- Burrs: 1.5, 2.0 mm
- PTCA: 3.5 x 20 mm @ 18 atm
- Stent: 3 x PS1535

A) This aorto-ostial RCA lesion* in an 84 year-old female was treated with rotastent. Atherectomy was used to increase vessel compliance and to facilitate stent implantation.

Treatment of aorto-ostial lesions is not an FDA-approved indication.

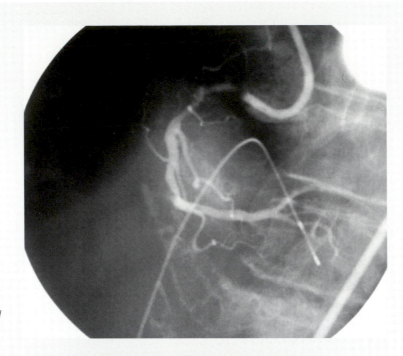

B) A 1.5 mm burr was initially used to treat the ostial lesion.

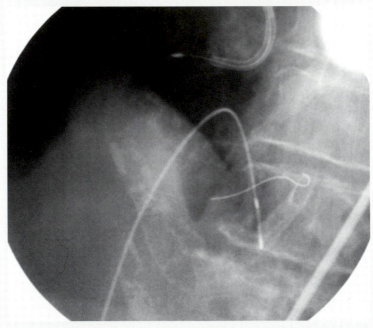

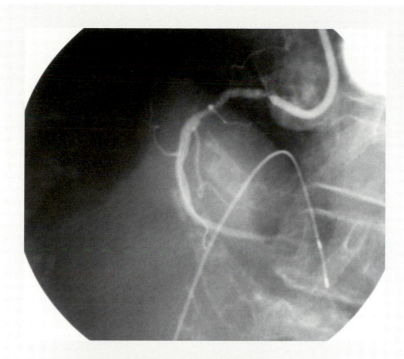

Figure 6.33 C&D
continued

C) Due to severe guidewire bias, a 2.0 mm burr ablation resulted in this hazy appearance at the lesion site. After PTCA, the lumen remained suboptimal and stents were placed.

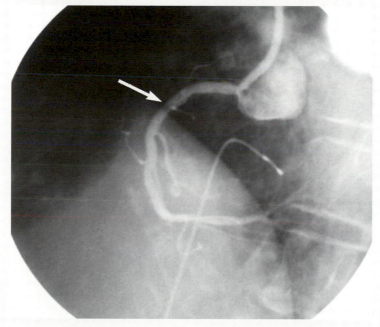

D) Three 3.5 mm stents were deployed to the ostium and proximal RCA. Post-stenting multiple balloon ruptures occurred, distal to the segment treated by the Rotablator (arrow). Retrospectively, this site should have been ablated prior to stent deployment. Intravascular ultrasound could have been used to better assess the significance and morphology of the disease beyond the ostium.

Figure 6.34 A-F

Stent for Dissection

Case Information:
- Guide Catheter: 8 Fr JL-4
- Guidewire: Type C
- Pacemaker: No
- Burrs: 1.5 mm, 2.0 mm
- PTCA: 3.0 mm @ 18 atms.
- Stent: 2 x PS1530

A) There are two high-grade proximal LAD stenoses (arrows) bridged by an ectasia in a moderately calcified LAD.

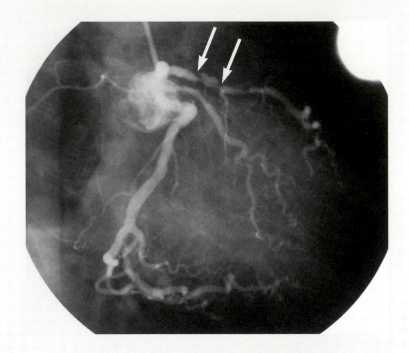

B) Note the "proximal" location of the guidewire to minimize guidewire bias and avoid vessel straightening in a tortuous distal vessel.

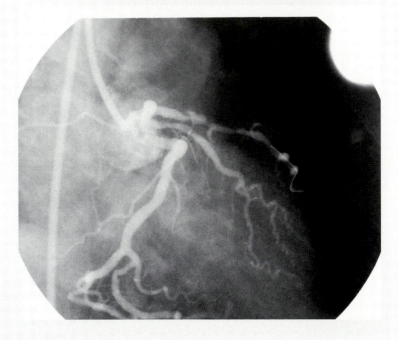

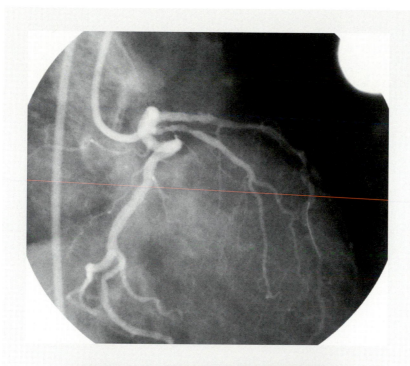

Figure 6.34 C&D
continued

C) The vessel was treated with 1.5 and 2.0 mm burrs.

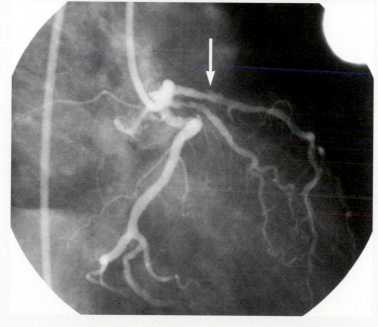

D) After PTCA at low pressure, there was a small dissection at the ectatic area (arrow) with evidence of recoil at the lesion site.

Figure 6.34 E&F
continued

E) The vessel continued to recoil with the dissection more apparent (arrow) despite further balloon inflations.

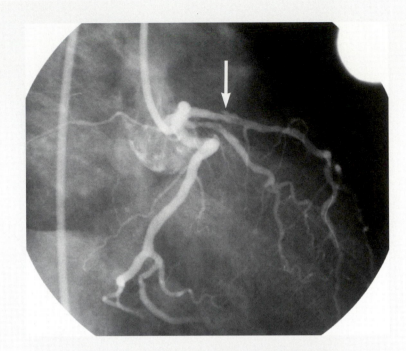

F) Two 3.0 mm stents were deployed, with complete coverage of the dissection and no residual stenosis.

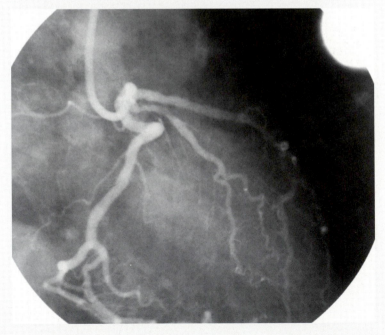

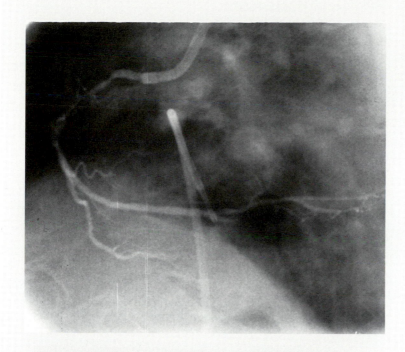

Figure 6.35 A&B

Rotastent of a Long Calcified Lesion

Case Information:
- Guide Catheter: 8 Fr JR-4
- Guidewire: Type C for RA, (Extra Support for stent)
- Pacemaker: Yes
- Burrs: 1.5, 1.75 mm
- PTCA: 3.0 x 20 mm, @ 18 atms.
- Stent: 2 x PS1530

A) A heavily calcified diffusely diseased RCA was treated with 1.5 and 1.75 mm burrs.

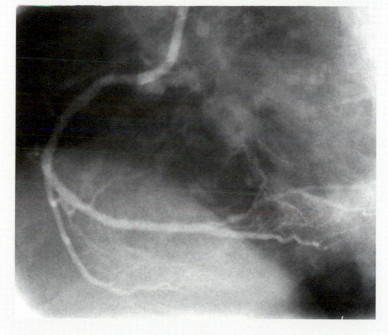

B) Two 3.0 mm stents were placed in the proximal and mid-vessel with an excellent result.

Intrastent Restenosis

The number of patients treated with intracoronary stents has increased dramatically over the last several years. In some catheterization laboratories 70–80% of patients having percutaneous interventions are receiving stents. Despite their impact in reducing restenosis, a significant number of patients will have recurrence of flow limiting obstructions at the stent site. The method of managing intrastent restenosis, which predominantly is a loss of lumen due to intimal hyperplasia, is under investigation.[59, 76, 77] Ablative strategies such as rotational atherectomy are appealing with the goal of increasing luminal dimensions by removing the neointimal tissue.

To date no reports have demonstrated "the downside" with the Rotablator system in fragmenting stent wires or inducing any acute complications. If the burr does make contact with the stent struts, they would be ablated into microparticles similar to inelastic

Figure 6.36 A-C

Treatment of Intrastent Restenosis

Case Information:
- Guide Catheter: 9 Fr JL-4
- Guidewire: Type C
- Pacemaker: No
- Burrs: 1.5, 2.0, 2.15 mm
- PTCA: 3.0 x 30 mm @ 4 atm
- Stent: Prior 1 x PS1530

A) This 64 year-old female had a stent placed in the LAD (arrow). Within 3 months it had restenosed and was treated with balloon angioplasty. She presented 3 months later with angina and intrastent re-restenosis.

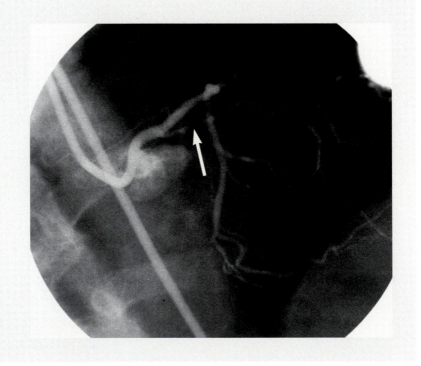

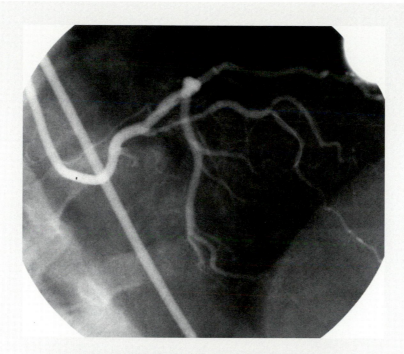

Figure 6.36 B&C
continued

B) The lesion was treated with 1.5, 2.0 and 2.15 mm burrs. Larger burrs were not used since the initial stent size (3.0 mm) was large for the artery, the plaque was present beyond the length of the stent, and guidewire bias was a concern.

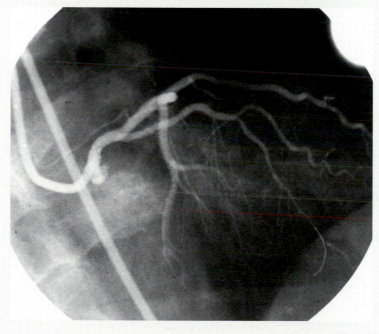

C) Instead of a larger burr, adjunctive PTCA was performed with a 3.0 x 30 mm balloon inflated at 4 atm.

Figure 6.37 A&B

Intrastent Restenosis

Case Information:
- Guide Catheter: 9 Fr JL-4
- Guidewire: Type C
- Pacemaker: No
- Burrs: 1.75, 2.25 mm
- PTCA: No
- Stent: Prior 1 x PS1530

A) This 44 year-old female with numerous risk factors had received a stent 7 weeks prior and returned with recurrent angina and a positive stress test. Intrastent restenosis was found in the LAD (arrow).

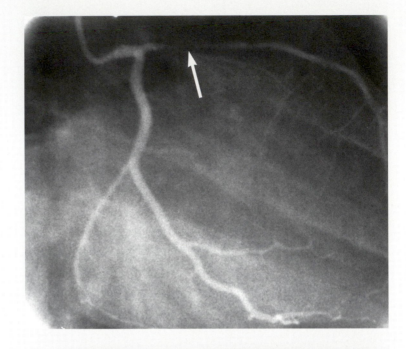

B) The lesion was treated with 1.75 and 2.25 mm burrs.

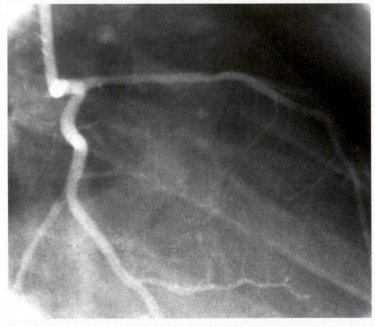

atherosclerotic plaque. The effects on the myocardium of the debris is presently the subject on ongoing research. The technique applied, which is still evolving, utilizes a step-approach with the final burr approaching 0.7–0.8 burr-to-stent ratio. Without adjunctive PTCA, generally a 3.0 mm stent is treated with a 1.75 mm burr followed by a 2.25 mm burr. Intravascular ultrasound has been shown to be helpful in defining the appropriate burr size.

Failed PTCA

Failed PTCA is either due to inability to cross the lesion or dilate. These lesions are frequently calcified. The timing to perform rotational atherectomy is determined by the lesion site after the attempted PTCA. If no dissection is evident angiographically, then there should not be a significantly increased risk to continuing with treatment by rotational atherectomy. If some luminal gain has been achieved with PTCA, beginning with a slightly larger burr can be considered. The technique and strategy should be managed as outlined in the preceding chapters.

Management of Complications

Chapter 7

Rotational atherectomy is associated with complications similar to other percutaneous procedures as well as some unique to this device. The interventional cardiologist and the entire catheterization staff should have a thorough understanding of these complications so that appropriate management can be expedited. This discussion will include: 1) atrioventricular block; 2) vasospasm; 3) slow flow and no reflow; 4) dissection; 5) perforations; 6) loss of side branches; 7) hypotension; and 8) thrombus.

Bradycardia and Atrioventricular Block

The incidence of bradycardia or atrioventricular block (AVB) is highest when treating lesions in the right coronary artery and left dominant circumflex with rotational atherectomy. AVB occurs occasionally in the LAD when large burrs (≥ 2.25 mm) are used to treat lesions at the ostium or proximal segment. The heart block can occur instantly after activating the device (more often in proximal lesions) or can follow a slowing trend. In both instances, the reestablishment of sinus rhythm can be achieved by deactivating the device.

The present recommendations are the placement of a temporary pacemaker in all patients undergoing treatment of the RCA, dominant left circumflex, and proximal LAD, and situations in which the treated lesion is collateralizing the RCA. The pacemaker is usually set at 50 bpm, to provide the benefits of atrioventricular synchrony at higher rates. The pacemaker should be tested prior to the procedure for assessment of ventricular capture. Blood pressure may drop more than expected when pacing and can indicate inadequate preoperative hydration. Pretreatment testing may afford an opportunity for this problem to be addressed.

Since coronary blood flow will be compromised during pacing, limiting run times during pacemaker activation is recommended.

The mechanism of bradyarrhythmia is unclear and theories have ranged from microparticles to microcavitations interfering with vessels perfusing the atrioventricular node. Another possibility is a yet-to-be understood reflex caused by vibrations or heat generated by the device.

It should be noted that several centers do not use temporary pacemaker wires. The patients are generally pretreated with atropine. Administration of atropine and maintenance of short ablation times can be beneficial to reduce the incidence of AVB. Their approach is to deactivate the device if slowing is noted. An alternate method of reestablishing sinus rhythm is to have the patient cough. Some centers advance the pacemaker only into the inferior vena cava and place it in the right ventricle when needed.

Since the AVB is transient, it is extremely rare for the patient to require the temporary pacemaker when leaving the cardiac catheterization laboratory.

Vasospasm

Coronary vasospasm used to be a frequent event during high-speed rotational atherectomy. With the routine use of a "rotaflush" (vasodilators placed in the infusate bag), the occurrence is greatly reduced.[62] Quantitative coronary angiography demonstrated that mild vasospasm occurred in reference segments and was relieved at the 24-hour post-procedure angiogram. The mechanism of vasospasm is unclear and there does not seem to be a greater predilection for one vessel. The precise incidence is unknown, but a potential trigger may be mechanical or a result of a blood product being liberated during ablation (e.g. from platelet activation). If vasospasm occurs, intracoronary nitroglycerin in moderate doses (150–200 mcgs) is beneficial. In addition, intracoronary calcium channel blockers (primarily verapamil at 100–150 micrograms doses) have been used. Bolus injections over a period of a few minutes in most cases are effective in breaking mild to moderate spasm. In more recalcitrant cases of vasospasm, vasodilators have been administered directly to the site via a balloon catheter or end hole subselective device (i.e. transfer catheter). In the latter cases, smaller doses should be used.

If the vasospasm is not responsive to pharmacological intervention due to a refractory vessel or concomitant hypotension, making the use of vasodilators prohibitive, PTCA at low-pressures can help mechanically increase the vessel lumen. In instances of diffuse spasm, which is not infrequent with the Rotablator system, care must be taken to ensure appropriate balloon sizing for the small, tapered distal vessels.

After severe spasm has been relieved with vasodilators, it is acceptable to continue rotational atherectomy, and step up to larger burrs. If low-pressure balloon inflations were required to relieve the spasm, close inspection of the vessel is recommended to ensure no dissections have occurred which would compromise further use of the Rotablator system.

Slow Flow Post High-Speed Rotational Ablation

Slow flow, and the more profound no reflow, represent the most challenging adverse sequelae.[80] Slow flow and no reflow are observed to some degree in 5% of patients undergoing treatment with the Rotablator system.[35] Slow flow is a diminution of flow by 1-2 TIMI grades from the baseline antegrade flow. No reflow is defined as the cessation of flow into the distal coronary circulation of the treated vessel.

No reflow is identified angiographically by a contrast dye column with a back and forth movement usually at or near the lesion site but not infrequently distal to this segment without clearance of the contrast material. The mechanisms of slow flow and no reflow are poorly understood and may be one or more of the following: excessive plaque burden, microparticulate aggregation, vasospasm, platelet activation or treatment of a vessel subtending a previously infarcted segment. A retrospective analysis of a subgroup of patients correlated the treatment of long de novo lesions, long ablation times and compromised myocardium in the subtended arterial zone to an increased incidence of slow flow.[35]

Recently, a tremendous amount of attention has been focused on the potential of platelet activation and subsequent aggregation as the culprit in flow disturbances after rotational atherectomy. Data accumulated so far supports the use of Reopro as a pharmacological adjuvant with the Rotablator system. Further research and analysis is required prior to recommending the use of platelet inhibitors.[55, 56] Regardless of the etiology, the final common pathway is compromised flow to the myocardium.

Figure 7.1 A-F

No Reflow

Case Information:
- Guide Catheter: 8 Fr JL-4
- Guidewire: Type C
- Pacemaker: No
- Burrs: 1.5, 1.75 mm
- PTCA: 2.5 x 20 mm @ 2 atm

A) This proximal LAD was heavily calcified and was tortuous distal to the lesion. After atherectomy, the vessel experienced no reflow.

In this preprocedure shot, note the vessel tortuosity. The lesion is difficult to see due to contrast blush in the aortic root.

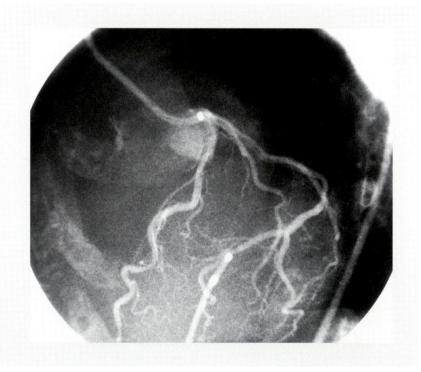

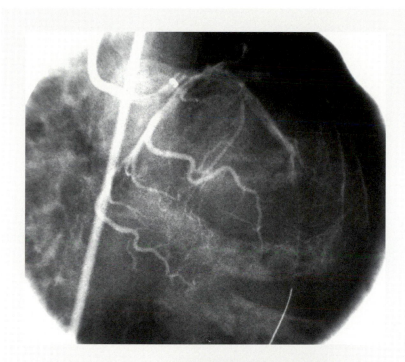

Figure 7.1 B&C
continued

B) No reflow occurred after atherectomy identified as stagnant flow distal to the lesion. This flow pattern would be atypical for dissection (see A).

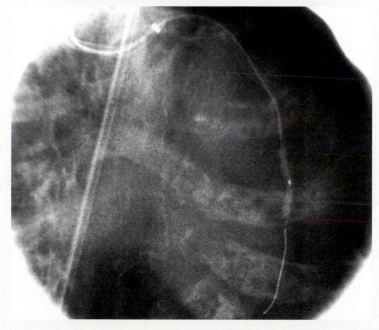

C) Despite treatment with nitroglycerin no flow persisted. PTCA was performed at low-pressure by "marching" the balloon in a distal to proximal fashion. (See D)

Figure 7.1 D&E
continued

D) Short (15 second) low-pressure (1–2 atm) inflations were used to restore flow. Note the more proximal location of the balloon compared to (C).

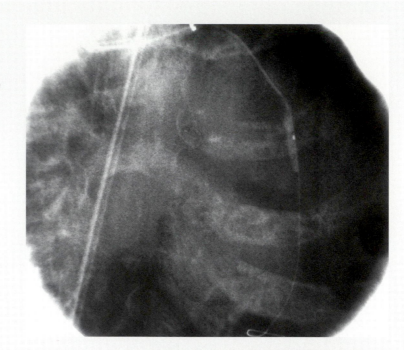

E) The final angiogram shows resumption of distal flow.

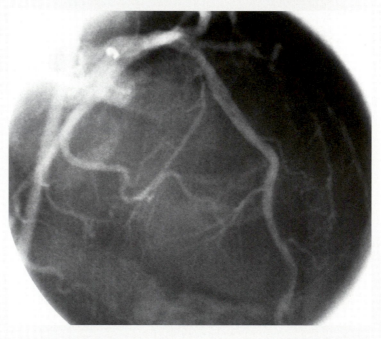

The ability to differentiate slow flow and no reflow from abrupt closure or flow-limiting dissection is important. Abrupt closure and flow-limiting dissections have distinctly different treatments than slow flow and no reflow. The cessation of flow due to abrupt closure from a severe dissection or flap should be treated with prolonged balloon inflations or stenting. In cases of abrupt closure the flow is compromised at the lesion site. The use of prolonged balloon inflations in the setting of slow flow (a non-structural complication) would not improve the situation and may accelerate a worsening clinical picture. In addition, severe vasospasm is sometimes difficult to differentiate from no reflow although the treatment is similar. Coronary vasospasm typically responds to vasodilators or low-pressure PTCA to "break" the spasm. Posttreatment, the vessel will regain baseline flow characteristics.

Slow and no reflow are managed in a similar fashion with the latter usually having a more deleterious hemodynamic impact, and therefore, requiring greater urgency. Slow flow and no reflow are usually noted after retracting the burr following a treatment. Once observed, no further ablation should be performed. The primary goal is to reduce the ischemic time. Initial steps include maintaining adequate perfusion pressure, either with aggressive hydration or vasopressors. If the patient does not respond adequately there should be no hesitancy to place an intra-aortic balloon pump. The intra-aortic balloon pump can frequently attend to the hemodynamics, and can also augment diastolic pressure which benefits the coronary blood flow.

Intracoronary nitroglycerin should be vigorously administered as tolerated either via the guiding catheter or through an end hole, subselective balloon, or transfer catheter. Other vasodilators such as verapamil have been used, but no single agent has demonstrated advantages over another.

The use of "blood" perfusion has also been an asset in these situations. Blood perfusion is performed by slowly withdrawing, blood from the sideholes of the guiding catheter into the manifold syringe and forcefully reinjecting the blood through the guiding catheter. Theoretically, high-pressure blood injections will accelerate particle clearance and perfuse the vessel.

Adjunctive balloon angioplasty is beneficial in these situations. To perform adjunctive PTCA, choose a balloon size that, at low pressure, will permit safe dilation beginning in the distal vessel. This will help to relieve vasospasm and the balloon may serve as a "plunger" to accelerate the egress of blood. ReoPro has also been used in cases with slow flow and, anecdotally, has been shown to be beneficial.

In summary, the management of slow flow or no reflow requires the integration of several techniques. The level of aggressiveness the operator needs with either pharmacological or mechanical intervention is typically mandated by the severity of the clinical parameters. Since slow flow and no reflow tend to worsen with time (a viscous cycle of low pressure causing further reduction in coronary flow), anticipate the possible deterioration and expedite therapy as quickly as possible.

Once flow has been reestablished, the electrocardiogram begins to normalize, but generally does not return to the baseline pattern even if all the epicardial vessels are well visualized. The patient's chest pain begins to improve, but usually requires time for complete resolution (approximately 20 minutes). A CPK elevation depends on the severity of the flow disturbance, and the amount of time that lapsed prior to its reconstitution.

Strategies to Reduce the Incidence of Slow and No Reflow
The following techniques and strategies should reduce the incidence of slow and no reflow.

Treatment strategies involve deploying burrs in a step method to minimize the effect of plaque burden for a given burr size. The technique of gentle advancement with intermittent retraction of the burr also decreases plaque burden. Gentle advancement minimizes the drop in rpm (no greater than 5,000 rpm), results in the smallest particle size, causes no significant generation of heat [20] and achieves appropriate plaque ablation for the burr used. The intermittent retraction of the device during ablation allows reestablishment of flow for particle clearance (see Figure 3.27).

Limiting ablation times to 15–30 seconds will decrease the plaque burden per unit of time. Increasing the time between ablations should also reduce the incidence of flow compromise. If an ablation is associated with significant chest pain with or without electrocardiographic changes, the time interval between treatment runs should be increased. The chest pain is felt to be secondary to compromised outflow in the distal microcirculation. Do not use a larger burr if no reflow or significant slow flow is present. Finally, platelet activation may be a significant contributor to flow compromise. Several retrospective clinical studies have shown a significantly lower CPK elevation with the administration of ReoPro when compared to Rotablator without platelet inhibitors in similar lesions.[80] Preliminary in vitro studies suggest that slower speeds (140,000–150,000 rpm) may reduce platelet aggregation and therefore may be beneficial.

Dissection

Angiographically visible dissections occur in approximately 10% of patients treated with the Rotablator system. Kovach et al. used sequential intravascular ultrasound and determined that after rotational atherectomy, 26% of patients had dissection planes. That number increased to 77% after adjunctive PTCA.[7] The location of dissection planes were predominantly within calcified plaque after rotational atherectomy and shifted to the vessel segment adjacent to the calcified plaque after adjunct balloon angioplasty.[7]

There are several mechanisms that have been implicated in Rotablator-induced dissections. When using appropriate step-burr sizing in a procedure, occasionally a dissection can be seen which does not stain or compromise distal flow following the use of the initial undersized device. Much debate has evolved over whether this situation represents an "underdone" result. The theory is that the surface of the plaque has been "unroofed" and that angiographic irregularities are the exposed inner aspects of the lesion, similar to splinters from a piece of wood.

This theory is consistent with the results reported by Mintz et al.[18] where 43% (12/28 pts) had fissures or dissections, and 29% had significant tissue disruption. When these dissections were assessed with intravascular ultrasound, they were typically superficial, located within the arc of calcified plaque, and had limited axial and circumferential extension. Dissections can be managed by deploying an oversized balloon at low pressures to "tack up the tissue". If larger burrs are considered, use of intravascular ultrasound is recommended.

In cases with moderate to severe angulation at the exit of the lesion, a trend toward increased dissections has been noted. This finding may be secondary to the stiffness of the guidewire, because in angles it does not follow the natural course of the vessel. The guidewire vector would cause the orientation of the burr to be out of plane, and result in tangential ablation with the potential of dissection.

Figure 7.2 A-C

Cap Dissection of RCA

Case Information:
- Guide Catheter: JR-4
- Guidewire: Type C
- Pacemaker: Yes
- Burr: 1.75 mm
- PTCA: 3.0 x 20 mm
  @ 4 atm, 4.0 x 20 mm
  @ 18 atm
- Stent: PS1535

A) There was a high-grade mid-RCA lesion. Comparison of the vessel with (A) and without (C) the guidewire demonstrates the guidewire straightening of the vessel.

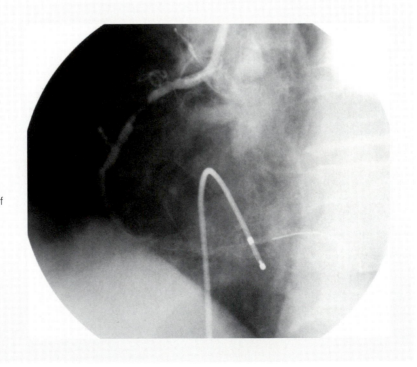

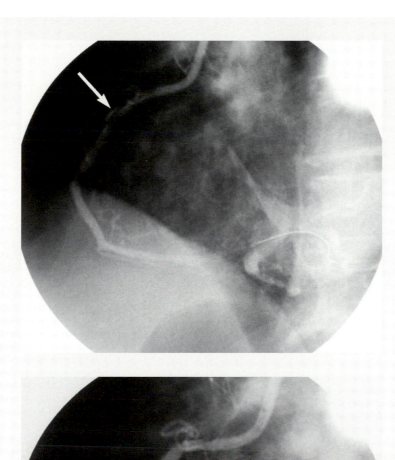

Figure 7.2 B&C
continued

B) After rotational atherectomy, the vessel appeared hazy and slightly disrupted. Post-PTCA, the dissection was apparent (arrow).

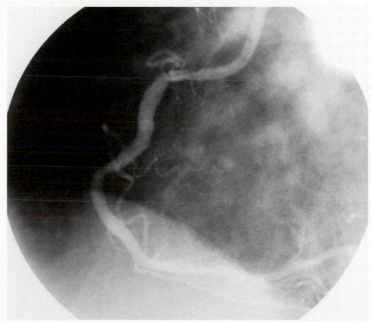

C) PS1535 was placed for treatment of the dissection.

Another site in which dissections appear to be more common is at the ostium of a severely angulated circumflex artery. Again, the stiffness of the wire can eccentrically orient the burr (due to guidewire bias) and force the burr to preferentially ablate on the inner aspect of the vessel. Therefore, in the case of an ostial circumflex on a severe bend, attempt to telescope the guide catheter to "remove" the angle. Amplatz guide catheters can be helpful. If improved alignment cannot be achieved, undersizing the burr for a maximum 0.5–0.6 burr-to-artery ratio and subsequently attempt to achieve the best result with adjunctive PTCA (lesion modification).

Rotablator dissections that are similar to angiographic complications with PTCA, involving large flaps and dye staining, should be handled with similar methods. If severe dissections occur, further ablation strategies should be avoided.

Figure 7.3 A-C

Flow-Limiting Dissection of Diagonal

Case Information:
- Guide Catheter: 9 Fr JL-4
- Guidewire: RotaWire Support
- Pacemaker: No
- Burrs: 1.75, 2.15 mm
- PTCA: 3.5 x 20 mm @ 2 atm & 16 atm
- Stent: 1 x PS1535

A) This 68 year-old male had multivessel disease with a 95% stenosis of the LAD at the takeoff of the first diagonal.

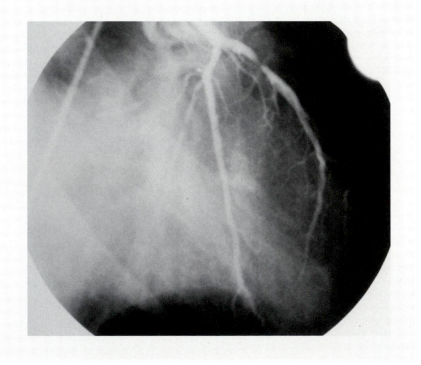

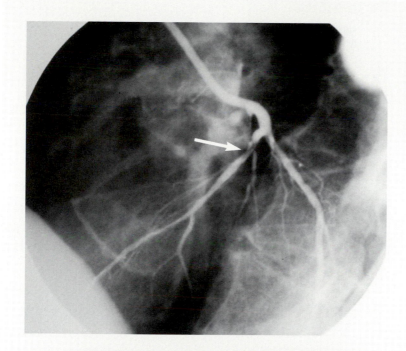

Figure 7.3 B&C
continued

B) After treatment with 1.75 and 2.15 mm burrs a small dissection or filling defect was noted opposite the diagonal artery (arrow). Treatment with adjunctive PTCA failed to resolve the defect and resulted in decreased flow to the diagonal artery.

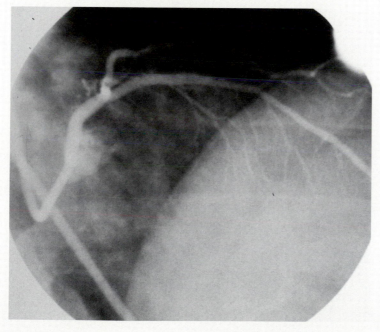

C) Attempts to cross the diagonal lesion with a guidewire failed. The dissection was treated with a 3.5 mm stent in the LAD, with sacrifice of the small diagonal.

Perforations

The incidence of perforation as reported from the multicenter registry was 0.7%.[81] The mechanisms for perforation include the use of oversized burrs, or a burr that is tangentially oriented due to the trajectory of the guidewire, denoted as unfavorable guidewire bias. The cause of perforation in cases of guidewire bias is most likely a result of the guidewire placing significant stress on the vessel wall. This will occur in severely angulated lesions (Figure 7.5 and Figure 7.6) or in vessels that are tortuous where the guidewire is directed preferentially (Figure 3.9) to one wall. This can occur even in cases where the vessel is elastic, since the strain or penetration of the guidewire into the wall will exceed the elasticity of the vessel and ablation of tissue will occur and potentially result in perforation.

Therefore the methods to avoid perforation are to minimize guidewire bias by guide catheter and guidewire placement and to

Figure 7.4 A-C

Perforation of Severely Angulated Vessel

Case Information:
- Guide Catheter: 8 Fr JL-4
- Guidewire: Type C
- Pacemaker: Yes
- Burr: 1.75 mm
- PTCA: 2.5 balloon, post-perforation

A) This severely angulated ostial stenosis of the obtuse marginal branch was treated with a 1.75 mm burr. A 1.75 mm burr is oversized since the risk of perforation is high, due to unfavorable guidewire bias. A smaller burr-to-artery ratio (0.5–0.6) with a strategy of lesion modification is recommended.

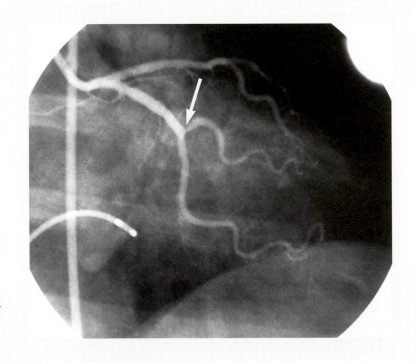

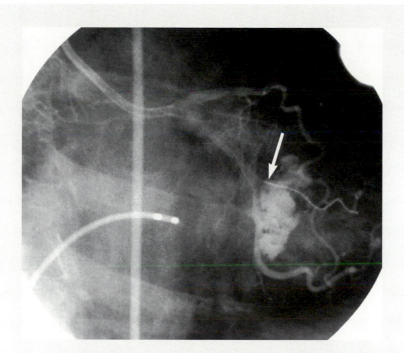

Figure 7.4 B&C

B) Treatment with a 1.75 mm burr resulted in this perforation (arrow). A smaller initial burr (1.5 mm maximum) and a "pecking" ablation technique should have been utilized. (See Chapter 6 on "Angulated Lesions", page 168.)

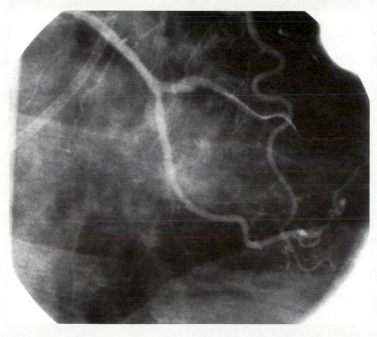

C) The perforation was treated with a perfusion balloon.

Figure 7.5 A-C

Perforation Due to Guidewire Bias

Case Information:
- Guide Catheter: 8 Fr JL-4
- Guidewire: Type C
- Pacemaker: Yes
- Burr: 1.5 mm
- PTCA: 2.5 x 30 mm

A) This 57 year-old male had a 99% stenosis of the LAD and an 80% focal stenosis in the circumflex.

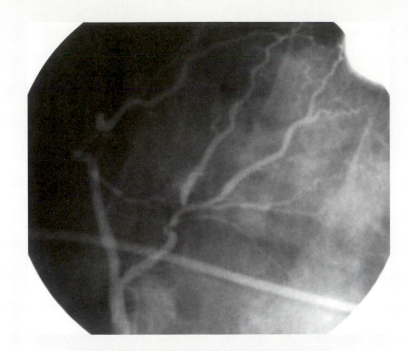

B) The guidewire vectored superiorly just distal to the bifurcation resulting in a perforation (arrow).

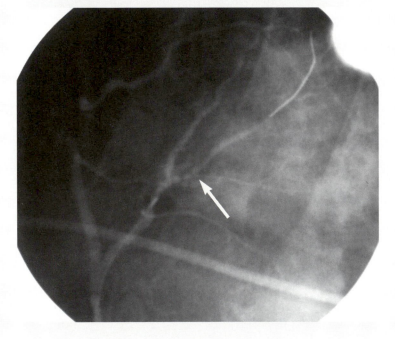

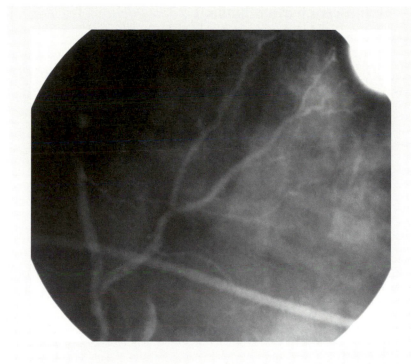

Figure 7.5 C
continued

C) The perforation was sealed with a 2.5 mm x 30 mm balloon at low-pressure (1 atm) for 5 minutes.

undersize the burrs (final burr-to-artery ratio of 0.6) in severely angulated or tortuous segments, especially those that are straightened by the guidewire or demonstrate the appearance of pseudolesions. In lesions that are severely angulated, a "pecking" technique should be applied to avoid excessive cutting to one wall, with the strategy of rotational atherectomy to improve vessel compliance for the adjunctive use of PTCA or other therapies. Another technique is to "relax" the guidewire prior to ablating. This method of removing the tension or the tethering effect (refer to Figure 3.10) may reduce the strain to the vessel wall.

Treatment of perforation is similar to those techniques standard to balloon angioplasty.

Side Branch Management

Since secondary or protecting wires for bifurcated lesions cannot be used with the Rotablator system careful attention should be paid to side branch management.[82] In most cases, side-branch occlusion during rotational atherectomy is a due to ablated microparticulate debris or vasospasm. In contrast, side-branch occlusion during PTCA, results from stretching the septum by inflating a balloon in one limb of the bifurcation, which impinges on the adjacent vessel and from plaque shifting.

When treating the left anterior descending, vasospasm may occur at the ostium of a diagonal or septal branch in the course of the ablation. In the right coronary artery, the problem usually involves small right ventricular branches that may be associated with minimal ECG and hemodynamic consequences, but can cause the patient profound chest discomfort. The vasospasm generally responds to vasodilators, and in the case of the diagonal artery, if it does not improve over a reasonable duration, performing low-pressure balloon inflation at the site of the spasm is sometimes worthwhile.

In cases of abrupt closure of a side branch after rotational atherectomy, treatment should be initially attempted with vasodilators.

One technique tip is to platform the burr distal to the takeoff of larger side branches if possible. This will reduce the possibility of inducing vasospasm.

The experience in treating bifurcation lesions that have disease in both arms is dependent on the sizes of the vessels (see Chapter 6 "Bifurcations" page 174). In treating bifurcation LAD/diagonal stenoses, the LAD and the larger diagonals are ordinarily ablated while the small diagonals are treated with PTCA. If the ostial diagonal is not dilatable with pressures of 4–6 atms, then an undersized burr is used to increase vessel compliance with subsequent adjunctive PTCA lesion modification.

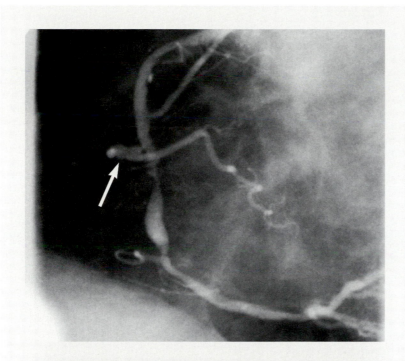

Figure 7.6 A&B

Loss of Side Branch

Case Information:
- Guide Catheter: 9 Fr JR-4
- Guidewire: Type C
- Pacemaker: Yes
- Burr: 1.5, 2.0 mm
- PTCA: 3.5 x 20 mm
  @ 2 atm

A) This 67 year-old male presented with exertional angina and had a 90% stenosis of the severely calcified RCA.

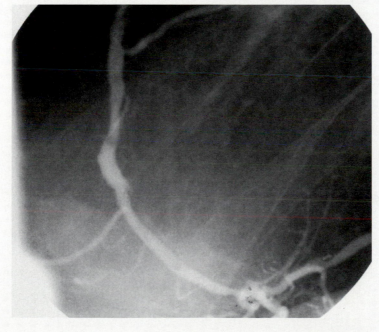

B) The lesion was treated with 1.5 and 2.0 mm burrs followed by a 3.5 mm balloon at 2 atm. The patient experienced moderate chest pain with no ECG changes or hemodynamic consequences. The right ventricular branch (see arrow in A) proximal to the lesion site has decreased flow due to vasospasm or no reflow and only a remnant of the vessel is visible.

Thrombus

Patients with evidence of angiographic thrombus have been generally excluded from treatment with the Rotablator system. In addition, patients with acute syndromes on admission have often undergone several days of anticoagulation prior to a Rotablator procedure. This approach is based on the soft substrate of a thrombotic occlusion and the limited value of the Rotablator on such an obstruction.

There are cases of thrombosis after the initial burr. In this situation, further use of the Rotablator should be based on the lesion characteristics. If the lesion is significantly calcified and it is felt that a balloon would be ineffective, then increasing to a larger burr would be acceptable. In general however, operators should not use larger burrs with the appearance of thrombus at a lesion and attempt to resolve the problem with PTCA, thrombolytics or recently available platelet inhibitors.

Hypotension

Hypotensive episodes exemplify the dichotomy between PTCA and rotational atherectomy. In PTCA the inciting factor is typically mechanical, such as a luminal disruption or dissection, and requires further balloon therapy, stenting, or, ultimately referral for bypass surgery. In Rotablator procedures the antecedents of the hypotensive episode can be vasospasm, slow or no reflow, bradycardia and, often, an inadequately hydrated patient receiving vasodilators. These events are frequently unpredictable and only with early recognition and expedient treatment can a deteriorating situation be reversed. Therefore, a well-prepared technical staff is fundamental in being able to address these issues.

Coronary blood flow is a major determinant of particle clearance. Therefore, starting the procedure with a low blood pressure is suboptimal. At the beginning of the procedure, the patient's volume status must be assessed and appropriately managed. If the patient is hypovolemic, the procedure should be delayed until fluids are administered. The use of large bore (7–8 Fr) venous sheaths can

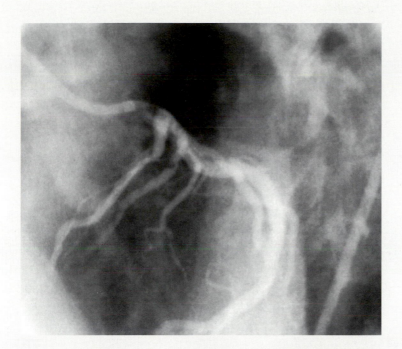

Figure 7.7 A&B

Thrombus

Case Information:
- Guide Catheter: 8 Fr JL-4
- Guidewire: HI-Torque Floppy exchanged for Type C
- Pacemaker: No
- Burr: 1.5, 2.0 mm
- PTCA: 3.0 x 20 mm @ 2 atm

A) This 52 year-old male was admitted for unstable angina and placed on heparin. He had an eccentric 90% stenosis of the LAD and a 90% stenosis of the diagonal. Both appeared to have calcium.

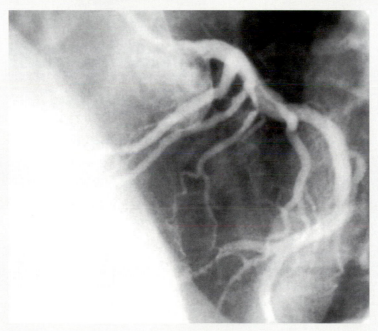

B) After a 1.5 mm burr there was sluggish flow in the distal LAD suggestive of thrombus. Flow was improved by vasodilators and since the vessel was known to be heavily calcified, a larger 2.0 mm burr was applied. Post procedure TIMI grade III flow was established with 15% residual stenosis. The diagonal was also treated with a 1.5 and 2.0 mm burrs followed by PTCA with less than 15% residual stenosis.

facilitate this process. The catheterization laboratory staff should have dopamine either mixed or easily accessible. For high-risk cases, an intra-aortic balloon pump should be available.

If intraprocedural hypotension occurs after ablation, infuse fluids. If the TIMI flow is reduced and the patient's overall status appears to be deteriorating, then do not hesitate to begin vasopressors, while the fluids infuse. If there is a question of volume status, a pulmonary artery catheter can be inserted.

In the situation of concomitant hypotension with slow or no reflow, an intra-aortic balloon pump is the therapy of choice.

Management of Rotablator System Failure

Despite the mechanical complexity of the Rotablator system, device failure is a rare event. In addition, the majority of device failures are generally secondary to use of the device outside the standard operations. The following section details the potential failures that could occur and their respective management.

Burr Detachment

There have been rare instances in which burrs have detached from the driveshaft cable. These detachments have usually been associated with significant force exerted to remove the nonspinning burr from the artery. To avoid this potential occurrence, do not use burrs that have less than 0.004" clearance for the guiding catheter. If the clearance is less than 0.004" then slow inactivated withdrawal of the burr is probably the best method to enter the guide catheter. In addition, when bringing the burr from the artery into the guiding catheter in preparation for an exchange procedure, verify that the guiding catheter is coaxial so that the burr doesn't get caught on the lip. If these suggestions are followed, the occurrence of detached burrs will remain rare.

If the burr detaches from the driveshaft cable, the distal tip of the guidewire (0.017" diameter) will keep the burr from exiting the end of the guidewire and the entire guiding catheter and guidewire system can be withdrawn. If the guidewire is difficult to retract with the burr-detached system, use intracoronary nitroglycerin to vasodilate the entire vessel which should ease the withdrawal of the system. If there is a proximal stenosis which does not allow the burr to be removed, use either a fixed-wire system or a coaxial over-the-wire system and perform balloon inflations for facilitated withdrawal of the burr.

Burr Stalling

The Rotablator is a low-powered rotary sander driven by air pressure. The burr can stall if there is significant resistance to burr rotation. Burr stalls are generally caused by one or more of the items listed below:

- Kinking of the air hose.
- Overtightening of the Y-connector.
- Burr-to-artery ratio exceeding 1.0.
- Aggressive advancement of the device into a tight lesion.
- Spasm in the platform zone may cause stalling. Intracoronary nitroglycerin may relieve the spasm.
- Operation without saline infusion.

Guidewire Fracture

Excessive rotation of the burr in one position especially in angulated or tortuous arteries can cause excessive wear on the guidewire and burr and result in fracture. When long ablation times are required, reposition the guidewire between runs. Another cause of guidewire fracture is the formation of a loop which fractures as the operator pulls on the wire to remove the loop. The following guidelines can minimize guidewire problems:

- Keep the guidewire out of small branches.
- Do not operate the advancer over a sharp bend or kink it in the guidewire.
- Reposition the guidewire frequently during excessively long ablations.
- Fasten the wireClip properly.
- Avoid prolapsing the guidewire tip.

- Inject contrast to demonstrate there is flow around the wire.

If wire fracture does occur, use one of the snare systems that are presently available from several manufacturers to retrieve the fractured guidewire.

Inability to Withdraw the Burr from the Vessel

Another infrequent event is the inability to withdraw the burr back across the lesion. This situation can occur if a burr slips across the lesion without adequate treatment of the site. The back portion of the burr does not contain diamond chips, and is therefore unable to ablate. In this situation do not attempt to pull or vigorously retract the burr, but use intracoronary nitroglycerin to test whether vasodilation will facilitate withdrawal. If required, balloon angioplasty can be used to achieve adequate luminal dimensions for withdrawal of the device.

Timing for Surgical Referral

Optimal timing for emergent bypass surgery is essential for maximum myocardial salvage. Coronary artery vasospasm and the slow reflow phenomenon are frequently amenable to time and to pharmacological and mechanical intervention. These issues must be recognized and not confused with severe dissection and abrupt closure and addressed as quickly as possible to avoid the need for surgery.

If the clinical status continues to deteriorate and the patient is unresponsive to the above-mentioned therapies, surgical intervention should be anticipated.

Cath Lab Personnel

To replicate the high success and low complications rates that have been achieved at the multicenter investigational sites, interventional cardiologists and the technical support staff must be prepared to expediently address complications that may occur during the course of treatment. For example, there should be an intravenous line dedicated for the infusion of a high volume of fluids. In addition, dopamine should be premixed or identified in the laboratory and a balloon pump should be available for emergency use. Several small syringes with nitroglycerin should be easily accessible in the event of vasospasm. A temporary pacemaker should be available for placement in the right ventricular apex. Trained personnel for this procedure should be accessible if a problem arises. Preparations such as those mentioned above will aid immensely in achieving successful outcomes.[83, 84]

Appendix

Advancer Components

The following appendix is a detailed reference on the Rotablator components and parts. This reference may be especially useful to cath lab staff who may assist during the procedure.

Advancer

The advancer (Figure 1) acts as a support for the air turbine and as a guide for the sliding elements which control burr extension. A brake within the advancer body is designed to hold the guidewire firmly during burr rotation to prevent the wire from spinning or moving. The air turbine uses compressed gas to generate the high rotational speeds necessary for ablation. Using compressed gas allows the use of low, inertial, mass-driving elements which can be quickly started and stopped. The Rotablator Advancer air hose is a small-gauge hose and is designed to be flexible, allowing convenient placement of the advancer.

Burr and Driveshaft

The diamond-coated burr consists of a tapered body coated with fine diamond chips (Figure 2). The burr is connected to a flexible helical shaft which has a central lumen that permits passage of the guidewire.

Sheath

The Teflon™ sheath is .058" (1.4 mm) in diameter and is beveled at the tip to allow easy passage in the vessel (Figure 2). The sheath

Figure 1

Rotablator Advancer

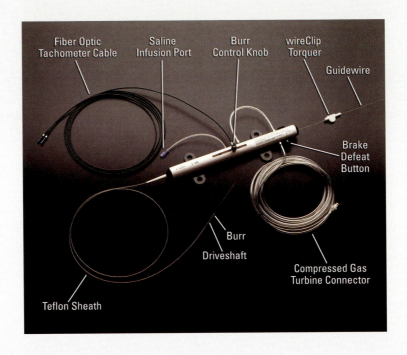

Fiber Optic Tachometer Cable · Saline Infusion Port · Burr Control Knob · wireClip Torquer · Guidewire · Brake Defeat Button · Burr Driveshaft · Compressed Gas Turbine Connector · Teflon Sheath

acts as a conduit to guide the helical drive from the point of entry to the site of the lesion, protects arterial tissue from the spinning driveshaft and permits the passage of saline to lubricate the driveshaft.

wireClip Torquer

The wireClip™ torquer is an accessory item provided in the pouch with the guidewire and is also available separately (Figure 3). The wireClip is side mounted on the guidewire by squeezing the two handles to open the clip jaws, placing the clip adjacent to the wire, and then moving the clip until the wire is entirely engaged in the groove of the clip. Releasing the handles will allow the wireClip to securely grasp the wire for steering or advancement. The clip can be repositioned as often as necessary. Always ensure that the wire is entirely engaged in the groove of the clip.

The wireClip prevents the guidewire from spinning when the

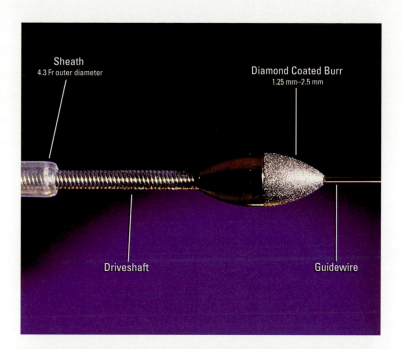

Figure 2

Rotablator Burr, Driveshaft and Sheath

Sheath
4.3 Fr outer diameter

Diamond Coated Burr
1.25 mm–2.5 mm

Driveshaft

Guidewire

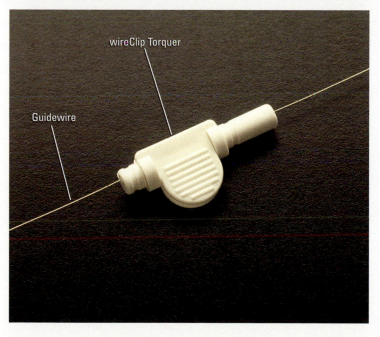

Figure 3

wireClip Torquer

wireClip Torquer

Guidewire

Figure 4

Schematic of Type C and Type A Guidewires

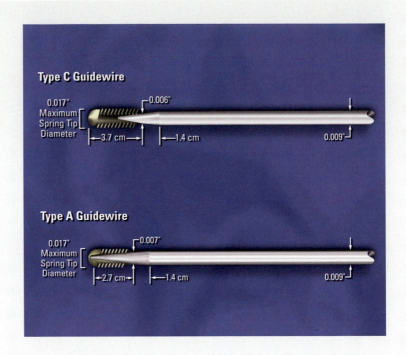

brake defeat is activated. It is also used as a torquing device. Never operate the guidewire break defeat unless you have a firm grip on the guidewire using the wireClip torquer. Defeating the brake without securing the guidewire may result in rotation and entanglement of the guidewire.

Guidewires

Initially two types of guidewires were available (Figure 4). The Type A has a diameter of .009" (0.23 mm), has a spring tip .017" maximum (0.43 mm) in diameter and 2.7 cm in length and a safety core that extends to the end of the spring tip. Type C is .009" (0.23 mm) in diameter and tapers at the distal end terminating in a flexible, formable platinum spring that is .017" maximum (0.43 mm) diameter and 3.7 cm in length. It contains a safety core that extends

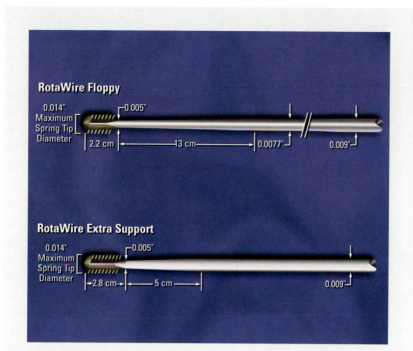

RotaWire Floppy

0.014"
Maximum
Spring Tip
Diameter

┌0.005"

2.2 cm   13 cm   0.0077"   0.009"

RotaWire Extra Support

0.014"
Maximum
Spring Tip
Diameter

┌0.005"

2.8 cm   5 cm   0.009"

to within 0.5" (12.71 mm) of the end of the spring. Both tip configurations render the wire atraumatic, improve the radiopacity of the devices, and can be preformed into a steerable system. The wire shaft of both guidewires is constructed of polished stainless steel. The wireClip™ torquer should be used to manipulate the wire.

RotaWire Guidewires

The recently released RotaWire guidewires (Figure 5) are designed to be more steerable and flexible than the earlier Type A and C wires. These improved handling characteristics are achieved by tapering the distal tip of the guidewire. In the RotaWire Floppy the taper begins further from the distal tip to increase flexibility. Both wires have short spring tips and the maximal

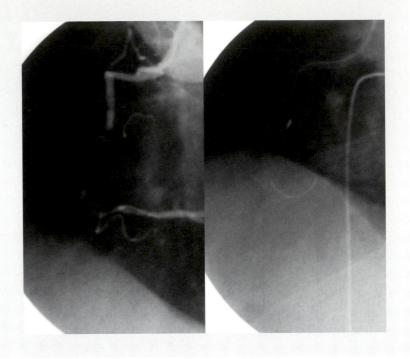

spring tip diameter is 0.014″ making it compatible with most balloon catheters.

The increased flexibility of the guidewire will reduce the side load tension of the guidewire against the wall of the artery reducing guidewire bias and will ease distal placement of the guidewire. The ability of the guidewire to follow the contours of a tortuous vessel can be seen in Figure 6.

Console Front Panel

The console (Figure 7 and 8) monitors and controls the rotational speed of the burr and continuously provides the operator with performance information during the procedure.

Power Switch

The push button power switch is located in the lower right corner of the front panel. The green light to the left of the switch illuminates

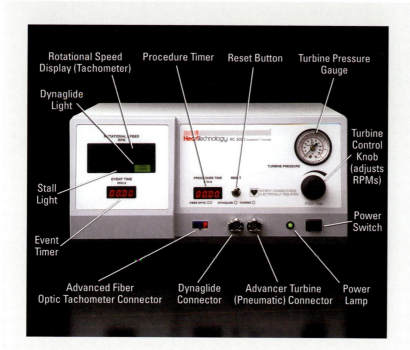

Figure 7
Front of Console

Rotational Speed Display (Tachometer)

Procedure Timer

Reset Button

Turbine Pressure Gauge

Dynaglide Light

Turbine Control Knob (adjusts RPMs)

Stall Light

Power Switch

Event Timer

Advanced Fiber Optic Tachometer Connector

Dynaglide Connector

Advancer Turbine (Pneumatic) Connector

Power Lamp

to indicate that the power has been turned on. Power is applied to the console when the switch is in the depressed position.

Turbine Control (Rotational Speed) Knob

A knob located above the power switch is used to adjust the gas pressure to the turbine and consequently, the rotational speed. Turning the knob clockwise increases the turbine pressure (speed) as indicated on the turbine pressure gauge. When the foot pedal is depressed, the rotational speed is shown on the appropriate front panel display.

Turbine Pressure Gauge

Located above the Turbine Control knob, the turbine pressure gauge displays the pressure of the compressed gas being supplied to the advancer gas turbine. Generally the greater the gas pressure to the gas turbine, the higher the rotational speed. The pressure should not be adjusted to exceed 70 psi (4.8 bar) during normal operation. Flow restrictions have been incorporated into the pneumatic system to prevent the delivery of excessive energy to the advancer.

Rotational Speed Display (Tachometer)

The rotational speed display located in the upper left corner of the console indicates the speed in rpm of the burr and gas turbine. When the gas turbine is not operating, the display is blank.

Stall Light

The stall light is located directly below the rotational speed display, and is visible only when illuminated. If the rotational speed of an advancer falls below 15,000 rpm for more than 0.5 seconds, the word "stall" is illuminated in red and delivery of compressed gas to the advancer is discontinued. A stall condition may also be detected if the fiber optic connection is not properly engaged. Stall detection is a safety feature designed to discontinue delivery of compressed gas to the advancer in the event of excessive mechanical loading or incorrect connection of the fiber optic. Releasing the foot pedal will clear the stall condition and extinguish the stall light.

Dynaglide Light

The dynaglide light is located adjacent to the "stall" light, and is visible only when illuminated (Dynaglide activated). Dynaglide provides a controlled low speed rotation (50,000–90,000 rpm) of the Rotablator burr for use during intraprocedure exchange of Rotablator advancer/catheters. The Dynaglide foot pedal button is used to turn Dynaglide on or off, and the word "Dynaglide" is illuminated in green when Dynaglide is activated.

Event Timer

Located below the tachometer, the event timer records how long the foot pedal has been continuously depressed with the air turbine and burr spinning. When the foot pedal is released, the timer continues to display the previous event time recording (the time during which the burr was spinning). Depressing the foot pedal resets and restarts the timer.

Procedure Timer

The procedure time is the sum of the individual event times and indicates the total time the burr has been spinning during the procedure.

Reset

Pushing the reset button resets the event and procedure timers to zero.

Advancer Turbine (Pneumatic)

The gas line connector on the right hand side receives the advancer gas hose and supplies filtered, regulated compressed gas to the advancer when the foot pedal is depressed.

Dynaglide Connector

The gas line connector on the left hand side receives the Dynaglide foot pedal red hose, and is used to activate or deactivate the Dynaglide.

Advanced Fiber Optic Tachometer Connectors

These two female connectors receive the mating male connectors from the fiber optic tachometer cable. The orientation of the cable to the female connector is not important. The fiber optic tachometer cable carries light pulses which the console uses to determine the gas turbine and burr speed.

Figure 8

Back of Console

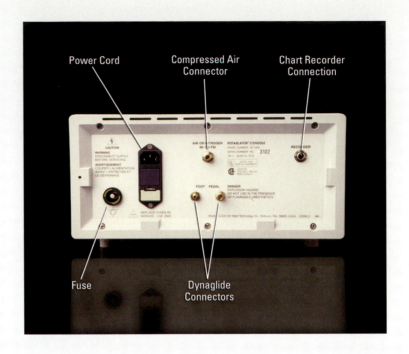

Console Back Panel

Outlined below are the main features on the back panel of the Rotablator console (Figure 8) and their functions.

Power Cord

This cable plugs into a conventional 120 VAC or 230 VAC receptacle (as indicated on the name plate located on the rear of the console) and provides power to the console.

Fuse

The fuse protects the console's electrical components in the event of a serious electrical fault. Located to the left of the fuse, a potential equalization connector is provided to allow potential equalization between various hospital electrical instruments.

Compressed Air Connector

This male connector, located in the top center of the rear panel, mates to the corresponding connector on the supply line from the compressed gas source. Pressure at this inlet should always be between 90 and 110 psi (6.5–7.5 bar) with a minimum flow capacity of 5 scfm (140 1/min). Pressure will be reduced by the console to operating limits. An internal pressure-relief valve protects against input pressures in excess of 115 psi (8.6 bar) and creates a loud hissing noise in the console if activated.

Dynaglide Connectors

These two connectors receive the mating pair of connectors from the Dynaglide foot pedal. The green hose connects to the right hand connector and the blue hose to the left hand connector.

Chart Recorder Connection

The recorder jack is used to connect a standard chart recorder or similar device to record the burr rotational speed over time. It may be used to assist with clinical training. It allows physicians who are newly trained on the Rotablator System to monitor the rpm changes throughout the procedure. The voltage output is 0.4V/100,000 rpm with an output impedance of 100 ohm.

Dynaglide Foot Pedal

The foot pedal (shown at the left in Figure 10) is used as an on/off control for the advancer gas turbine . The foot pedal is also fitted with a valve which vents any compressed gas in the foot pedal hose when the pedal is released, permitting rapid stopping of the burr. The foot pedal is mounted in a protective shroud which inhibits accidental start-up.

The Dynaglide button located on the right side of the foot pedal housing is used as an on/off control for the Dynaglide mode of operation. When Dynaglide is on, the green "Dynaglide" light is illuminated on the console front panel.

Figure 9

Exchangeable Driveshaft

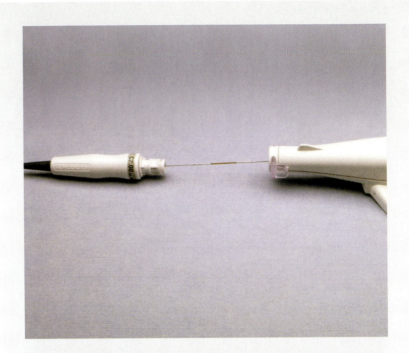

Figure 10

Rotablator System with Exchangeable Driveshaft

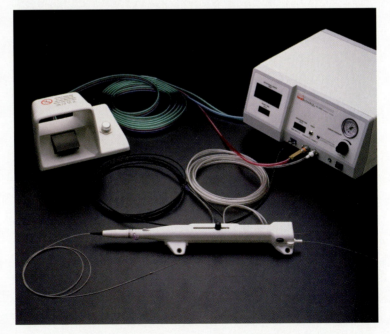

Exchangeable Driveshaft

The exchangeable driveshaft was designed to simplify the Rotablator procedure, both in terms of cost and reduced time in the catheterization laboratory. The new design allows the operator to replace only the driveshaft portion of the advancer during a procedure (Figure 9). This component design allows one advancer housing to be used with several different burrs. In procedures that require the use of multiple burrs a substantial time and cost savings can be realized. This advance over the old design enhances the competitiveness of the Rotablator system relative to other interventional therapies. This is especially important in today's cost-conscious health care environment.

The exchangeable driveshaft is being introduced to the interventional community in 1997.

Rotablator Assembly Procedure

(For complete instructions for the assembly and operation of the Rotablator system, refer to the Operator's Manual.)

Prior to Procedure

1) Acquire a compressed gas cylinder containing either compressed air or nitrogen. A cylinder capacity of at least 80 standard cubic feet 2,250 liter is recommended, and will provide approximately 20 minutes of service with the Rotablator Advancer running at full speed. Larger cylinders may be used, and a fully charged spare cylinder should always be available. Secure the compressed gas cylinder by strapping it firmly to a cart, wall bracket, or table clamp per hospital protocol.

2) Obtain a cylinder pressure regulator (relieving type is preferred) capable of delivering at least 5 scfm (140 liter/min) at 90–110 psi (6.5–7.5 bar). Make certain that the regulator's cylinder fitting is compatible with the gas cylinder being used and that the supply hose gas coupling provided with the Rotablator console is compatible with the outlet port of the regulator or that an adapter is available.

3) Remove the cylinder cap and attach the regulator, tightening the cylinder fitting firmly. The regulator should be adjusted so that the outlet pressure is in the range of 90–110 psi (6.5–7.5 bar). If the pressure in the tank is below 900–1000 psi consider changing tanks before the procedure begins.

At the time of the procedure:

4) Connect the supply hose between the regulator and the inlet connector on the back of the console.

5) Connect the foot pedal to the console by locating the three connectors at the end of the foot pedal triple hose. Insert the green hose connector in the right side and the blue hose connector in the left side mating receptacles on the rear of the Rotablator console. These receptacles are labeled "Foot Pedal" or marked with a foot pedal symbol. The red hose connector is connected to the left hand connector on the front panel.

6) Connect the power cord to a properly rated hospital grade receptacle (as indicated on the nameplate located on the rear of the console). Push the console power switch and confirm that the green power indication light illuminates.

During the Procedure: Guidewire Assembly and Placement

7) Position a guiding catheter or sheath in the vessel of interest. Verify that the intended catheter has an adequate internal lumen diameter to pass the largest burr to be used. The guiding catheter selected should have an internal diameter of 0.004" greater than the burr in order to comfortably accommodate the burr.

   The guiding catheter can be placed using conventional catheterization techniques. A hemostasis valve with side port or a "Y" adapter may be placed on the guide catheter hub to prevent back bleeding, and its side port can be used for contrast injection. When using guide catheters with "Y" adapter, be aware that the hemostasis valve may permit insertion of the burr, but inhibit or prevent its retraction. Always check compatibility of burrs and hemostatic devices before insertion.

Some hemostasis valves can inhibit or prevent retraction of the burr.

8) Guidewires are provided separately in a sterile pouch with a chevron seal. The wireClip torquer is packaged with the guidewire and can be found on a holding card.

9) Select a guidewire appropriate for this procedure.

10) Open the peel pouch, and using sterile technique, extract the coil. The distal tip of the wire is located in the inside blue cap.

11) Remove the inside (proximal) cap, grasp the wire with fingers or a wireClip torquer, and slowly remove the wire. The wire is coated with a thin film of lubricant and exhibits a slight drag as it is extracted from the coil. If there is difficulty removing the wire, remove the tube clips and straighten the packaging tube.

12) Attach the wireClip to the proximal end of the guidewire and gently pull from the packaging tube.

13) Lubricant may be visible on the guidewire. This lubricant in no way compromises the use of the guidewire. Use care not to stretch or damage the spring tip. The guidewire must be handled carefully. A tight loop, kink, or sharp bend (greater than 90°) in the guidewire may cause it to fracture during use.

14) Thread the guidewire into the hemostasis valve and guide catheter. Use a standard guidewire introducer tool with the guidewire. It may be left in place, with the hemostasis valve tightened around it, while the guidewire is steered across the lesion. The introducer tool must then be backed off the guidewire before the Rotablator advancer/catheter is loaded onto the wire.

15) Attach the wireClip torquer to the guidewire. The wireClip torquer is packaged with the guidewire on a holding card in the guidewire pouch. The wireClip is side mounted on the guidewire by squeezing the two handles to open the clip jaws, placing the clip adjacent to the wire, and then moving the clip until the wire is entirely engaged in the groove of the clip. Releasing the handles will allow the wireClip to securely grasp

the wire for steering or advancement. The clip can be repositioned as often as necessary. Always ensure that the wire is entirely engaged in the groove of the clip.

Using standard angioplasty procedures, and under fluoroscopic guidance, gently advance the wire past the lesions using a bare-wire or free-wire technique. The wire spring tip must be placed distal to the lesion. Avoid placing the guidewire tip in a smaller side-branch artery.

16) In cases where the Rotablator guidewire is not sufficiently flexible or steerable, it is recommended to place a conventional commercial angioplasty guidewire in the artery first and guide it past the lesion. Then a small diameter exchange catheter can be placed over the wire, and the wire exchanged for the Rotablator guidewire. The Rotablator catheter can then be threaded over the Rotablator guidewire to the site of the lesion.

17) Due to the fact that the Rotablator system is an over-the-wire coaxial device, it is possible to form loops in the guidewire. Loops in the guidewire most frequently occur when the guide catheter is inadvertently disengaged from the ostium. The formation of a loop may also occur if inadequate tension is placed on the guidewire as the burr is being advanced over the wire. If there is a loop in the guidewire, do not pull on the wire to straighten it as this action may cause the wire to fracture. To remove a loop from the guidewire, first pull back slightly on the guide catheter. With the guide catheter out of the ostium, rotate the guidewire one-half turn counterclockwise to remove the loop. If the loop still exists, rotate the wire one-half turn in the other direction and reevaluate. With the loop removed, re-seat the guide catheter while pulling back on the guidewire. Any time a loop in the guidewire is seen, it is important to note that merely pulling back on the wire will not safely remove the loop. The optimal method for removing a loop in the guidewire is to rotate the wire as outlined above.

Advancer and Burr Preparation

18) After the Rotablator guidewire is selected and in place distal to the lesion as described, select the appropriate burr size (refer to Chapter 3 "Burr Selection", page 70).

19) The Rotablator advancer/catheter is double packaged so that the complete kit, including tray, can be placed in a sterile field. Open the Rotablator advancer/catheter shelf box, remove the sheet of protective foam, and lift out the tray in its sterile pouch. Peel the corner of the sterile pouch until the majority of the tray is exposed. Inverting the pouch will now allow the tray to slide out onto a sterile drape, or, alternatively, a person using sterile technique can pull the tray from the pouch and place it on a sterile drape.

20) To expose the advancer, peel away the lid using the gray pull tab provided, revealing the inverted advancer inside. Locate and discard the small foam blocks which retain the catheter in its grove. Using one hand to restrain the advancer, gently invert the tray onto the drape, and then lift and discard the tray. The advancer will now be resting on its feet. Locate the end of the catheter and position it in the direction of the treatment or entry site. Remove the red tie from the advancer hose by pulling the finger ring. Uncoil the hose and pass it out of the sterile field towards the console. Have nonsterile circulating personnel connect the quick-disconnect to the properly sized receptacle labeled "Turbine" on the front of the console (Figure 7).

21) Identify the black fiber optic tachometer cable, and not the plastic connectors on its end. Remove the red tie by pulling the finger ring, uncoil the fiber optic tachometer cable and route it out of the sterile field towards the console. Have nonsterile circulating personnel insert the fiber optic connectors into the receptacles labeled "Fiber Optic" on the front of the console until they snap securely into place.

22) Using sterile technique, attach an infusion set to administer normal saline, and connect it to the infusion port on the

advancer. The saline should be pressurized with an IV pressure bag to ensure steady infusion against arterial pressure. The recommended pressure is 150–200 mm Hg.

23) Wait until the saline flows through the advancer and sheath, and exits from the sheath tip running bubble free. The seals of the advancer are designed to slowly weep saline. The weeping of saline is normal and does not indicate a malfunctioning device.

24) Always ensure either visually or by using an IV drip monitor that there is a free flow of saline from the distal sheath before operating the advancer. A small infusion pump incorporated into the advancer boosts the infusion pressure and flow rate when the air turbine is running. Never operate the Rotablator advancer without saline infusion. Flowing saline is essential for cooling and lubricating the working parts of the advancer and catheter. Operation of the advancer without proper saline infusion may result in permanent damage.

25) The Rotablator rotational angioplasty system is now ready for use.

Testing the System Prior to Use:

The Rotablator system must be tested before inserting the burr into the guiding catheter or sheath. The following summary is covered in more detail in the operator's manual. Please refer to it for more complete instructions.

26) With the guidewire in place distal to the lesion, grasp the proximal tip of the guidewire and thread this end into the hole in the tip of the burr. Continue feeding the wire into the catheter until it appears at the rear of the advancer, then grasp the exposed wire and pull it gently until the burr is a few centimeters from the guide catheter/ hemostasis valve. Remove any lubricant that may have built up on the burr during the guidewire loading by gently wiping with a gloved fingertip. Attach the wireClip torquer to the guidewire a few

centimeters behind the end of the advancer.

27) Depress the Dynaglide button on the foot pedal several times. Note that the green Dynaglide indicator on the console is alternately illuminated and extinguished. Push the Dynaglide button so that the indicator is extinguished.

28) Verify that the catheter tip is in free air and that the burr and guidewire are not touching any objects. Turn the turbine pressure adjustment knob fully counterclockwise so that the burr will not spin if the foot pedal is accidentally depressed. Always ensure that there is free flow of saline before operating the advancer.

29) Place the advancer in a fully retracted position. Hold the guidewire distal to the burr and the distal sheath to provide support for the burr. Rotate the turbine pressure knob to obtain a pressure gauge reading of 40 psi. Fully depress the foot pedal and adjust the pressure knob until the burr is spinning at the correct speed. Release the foot pedal. If the device does not run and the stall light is illuminated, release the foot pedal and check all advancer connections before trying again.

30) After setting the speed, practice advancing the burr while it is rotating. Slowly advance the burr knob and verify the corresponding advance of the burr along the guidewire.

31) With the system rotating grasp the wireClip torquer and attempt to retract the guidewire where it exits the back of the advancer. The wire should be firmly gripped by the internal automatic brake.

32) The burr and drive shaft will tend to whip if they are not confined to the lumen of a sheath. When operating the system outside the body always support the guidewire. Also note the drip rate of saline which should increase when the system is running. After the successful completion of these checks the system is ready to be advanced to the lesion.

Recommended Rotablator Advancer Turbine Speed

Burr Size (mm)	Rotational Speed Range (rpm)	Platform Speed (rpm)
1.25	150,000–190,000	180,000
1.5	150,000–190,000	180,000
1.75	150,000–190,000	180,000
2.0	150,000–190,000	180,000
2.15	140,000–180,000	160,000
2.25	140,000–180,000	160,000
2.50	140,000–180,000	160,000

Rotablator Catheter Sheath O.D.

Size: mm	Size: Fr	Size: Inches
1.35	4.0	0.058

Coronary Rotablator System Burr Size

Burr Size (mm)	Cross Sectional Area (mm²)	Guide Catheter Min. ID*
1.25	1.23	.053"
1.50	1.77	.063"
1.75	2.40	.073"
2.00	3.14	.083"
2.15	3.63	.089"
2.25	3.97	.093"
2.38	4.45	.098"
2.50	4.91	.102"

* The minimum internal diameter of the guide catheter should equal or exceed the number dimension listed.

Percent Increase of Cross-Sectional Area of Second Burr Compared to First Burr

First Burr (mm)	Second Burr (mm)						
	1.50	1.75	2.00	2.15	2.25	2.38	2.50
1.25	44	95	155	195			
1.50		36	77	105	124		
1.75			31	51	65	85	105
2.00				16	26	42	56
2.15					9	23	35
2.25						12	24
2.38							10
2.50							

Burr-to-Artery Ratio

Ref. Vessel DM (mm)

Ref. Vessel DM (mm)	Burr Size (mm)							
	1.25	1.50	1.75	2.00	2.15	2.25	2.38	2.50
2.00	.63	.75	.88					
2.25	.56	.67	.78	.89				
2.50	.50	.60	.70	.80	.86	.90	.95	
2.75	.45	.55	.64	.73	.78	.82	.87	.91
3.00	.42	.50	.58	.67	.72	.75	.79	.83
3.25	.38	.46	.51	.62	.66	.69	.73	.77
3.50	.36	.43	.50	.57	.61	.64	.68	.71

Summary of Articles on Rotational Atherectomy

Abbo KM, Dooris M, Glazier S, et al. Features and outcome of no reflow after percutaneous coronary intervention. Amer J Cardiol. 1995; 75(12):778–82. *Among 10,676 coronary interventions performed between October, 1988 and June, 1993, no reflow occurred in 66 patients (0.6%). The incidence of no reflow was 30 of 9,431 (0.3%) for percutaneous transluminal coronary angioplasty, 1 of 317 (0.3%) for excimer laser, 8 of 104 (7.7%) for RA, 21 of 469 (4.5%) for extraction atherectomy, and 6 of 355 (1.7%) for directional atherectomy. Those patients with no reflow, experienced a tenfold higher incidence of in-hospital death (15%) and acute myocardial infarction (31%). Correlates of in-hospital mortality included acute myocardial infarction on presentation (p = 0.006) and final flow < 3 (as defined by the TIMI trial) at completion of the procedure (p = 0.03).*

Abhyankar AD, Vaidya KA, Bernstein L. Rotational atherectomy of calcified ostial saphenous vein graft lesion with long term follow-up: A case report. Internat J Cardiol 1995; 52(1):11–2. *RA, though widely used for calcified and difficult lesions, has not been used in vein graft lesions. The study reported RA on a 75 year-old male with a calcified ostial lesion in an 11 year-old vein graft. No complications were encountered and good result was obtained. An angiogram at 10 months revealed no restenosis.*

Ahn SS, Auth D, Marcus DR, et al. Removal of focal atheromatous lesions by angioscopically guided high-speed rotary atherectomy: preliminary experimental observations. Journal of Vascular Surgery, 1988; 7:292–300.

Borrione M, Hall P, Almayor Y, et al. Treatment of simple and complex coronary stenosis using rotational ablation followed by low pressure balloon angioplasty. Cathet Cardiovasc Diag 1993; 30(2):131–7. *In the 166 patients treated with RA and low pressure PTCA, 63% with complex lesions, the clinical success was 100% for type A, 95% in B1, 98% in B2 and 93% in type C lesions.*

Left ventricular dysfunction, total occlusion and severity of stenosis were predictive of clinical failure. There were 3 deaths, 1 Qwave MI and 14 non-Qwave MIs.

Bowles M, Palko W, Beaver C, et al. Clinical and postmortem outcome of "no reflow" phenomenon in a patient treated with rotational atherectomy. Southern Med J. 1996; 89(8):820–3. *Postmortem evaluation of a patient who died after RA revealed atheroemboli in the myocardial arterioles of the distal bed.*

Bowling L S, Guarneri E, Schatz PA, et al. High-speed rotational atherectomy of tortuous coronary arteries with guidewire-associated pseudostenosis. Cathet Cardiovasc Diag 1996; Supple Summary 3:82–84.

Brogan WCD, Popma JJ, Pichard A, et al. Rotational coronary atherectomy after unsuccessful coronary balloon angioplasty. Amer J Cardiol 1993; 71(10):794–8. *This is a study of 41 patients (50 lesions) referred after an unsuccessful PTCA. RA reduced stenosis from 72 ± 14% to 41 ± 16%. Adjunct PTCA in 44 lesions reduced stenosis to 25 ± 17%. Angiographic success was obtained in 49 (98%) lesions. Procedural success (angiographic success without complications) was obtained in 37/41 procedures (90%).*

Cardenas JR, Strumpf RK, Heuser RR. Rotational atherectomy in restenotic lesions at the distal saphenous vein graft anastomosis. Cathet Cardiovasc Diag. 1995; 36(1):53–7. *RA was used to successfully treat the distal saphenous vein graft anastomoses in three patients with nonthrombotic focal restenosis of the vein graft touchdown.*

Chaix AF, Barragan P, Silvestri M, et al. Rotablator and endoprosthesis on the left main coronary trunk. [French] Archives des Maladies du Coeur et des Vaisseaux. 1995; 88(1):95–7. *This report describes the successful treatment by RA + angioplasty of the left main, LAD, and circumflex in a 78 year-old woman.*

Cohen BM, Weber VJ, Blumm RR, et al. Cocktail attenuation of rotational ablation flow effects (CARAFE) study: Pilot. Cathet Cardiovasc Diag 1996; Supple 3:69–72. *An infusion cocktail of verapamil, nitroglycerin and heparin was used in 27 lesions. In these procedures there were two cases of vasospasm and one transient slow flow occurrence. This incidence of slow flow (4%) is less than published reports (9%).*

Cohen BM, Weber VJ, Reisman M, et al. Coronary perforation complicating rotational ablation The US multicenter experience. Cathet Cardiovasc Diag 1996; Supple 3:55–59. *The study analyzed the incidence of coronary perforation in the multicenter registry of 2,953 procedures. There were 22 (0.7%) perforations. Of these 15 experienced a major complication including death 2, MI 6, surgery 9 or tamponade and 7 sealed with balloon angioplasty without sequelae. Perforations occurred more frequently in lesions which were long, eccentric or tortuous.*

Danchin N, Cassagnes J, Juilliere Y, et al. Balloon angioplasty versus rotational angioplasty in chronic coronary occlusions (the BAROCCO study). Amer J Cardiol. 1995; 75(5):330–4. *One hundred consecutive patients with total coronary occlusion were randomized to either RA or conventional angioplasty. The primary success rate in the RA group was 66% compared with 52% in the angioplasty group. In chronic coronary occlusions of tapered morphology, rotational angioplasty is not superior to conventional angioplasty. In stump-like occlusions, the primary success rate is higher with the rotational angioplasty technique.*

Deelstra MH. Coronary rotational ablation: an overview with related nursing interventions. American Journal of Critical Care 1993; 2(1):16–25; quiz 26–7. *A review of the Rotablator procedure and an outline of the nursing procedures associated with it.*

DeFranco AC, Nissen SE, Tuzcu M, et al. Incremental value of intravascular ultrasound during rotational coronary atherectomy. Cathet Cardiovasc Diag 1996; Supple 3:23–33. *This review of the use of ultrasound with rotational atherectomy suggests that preprocedure use may help direct the most appropriate choice of interventional modalities and confirms the smooth round lumen created by rotational atherectomy.*

Dietz U, Erbel R, Rupprecht HJ, et al. High-frequency rotational ablation following failed percutaneous transluminal coronary angioplasty. Cathet Cardiovasc Diag 1994; 31(3): 179–86. *After PTCA failed in 29 of 1,150 patients after successful passage of the guidewire, the RA was successfully used. Diameter stenosis was reduced from 87 ± 15% (including 14 chronic total occlusions) to 51 ± 18% post-RA to 41 ± 14% post-procedure (including PTCA in 21/29) to 36 ± 13% at 24 hrs post-procedure. The procedure was a success at 24 hrs in 26/29 (90%) of patients. No major complications occurred.*

Dietz U, Erbel R, Pannen B, et al. Angiographic and histologic findings in high-frequency rotational ablation in coronary arteries in vitro. [German] Zeitschrift fur Kardiologie 1991; 80(3):222–9. *The authors examined arteries after in vitro RA in humans and pigs. In humans the inner most layers were removed with frequent tears. 13/17 had tears, 3/17 medial tears. There was very little effect on the artery adjacent to the lesion.*

Dietz U, Erbel R, Rupprecht HJ, et al. High-frequency rotational ablation: An alternative in treating coronary artery stenoses and occlusions. British Heart J 1993;70(4):327–36. *This study describes the treatment of 106 patients, 67 with significant stenoses and 47 with chronic occlusions. In 5 stenoses and 15 chronic occlusions the guidewire was unable to cross the lesion. In 4 cases RA failed. When combined with balloon angioplasty success was achieved in 79% of the stenoses and 54% of the chronic occlusions. At six months restenosis was evident in 9/25 (36%) treated with RA alone, 7/22 (32%) treated with RA + PTCA and 14/24 (58%) chronic occlusions. Procedural complications included (2) CABGs, (0) deaths, (0) Qwave MI and (5) non-Qwave MI. Severe spasm unresponsive to medical therapy occurred in 7 cases.*

Dussaillant GR, Mintz GS, Pichard AD, et al. Mechanisms and immediate and long-term results of adjunct directional coronary atherectomy after rotational atherectomy. J Amer Coll Cardiol. 1996; 27(6):1,390–7. *To examine the synergistic relationship between rotational atherectomy and directional coronary atherectomy in the treatment of calcified lesions, 165 lesions treated with RA + DCA were compared to 208 lesions treated with RA + angioplasty. The immediate results showed a high procedural success — lumen dimensions were larger and late target-lesion revascularization was lower in lesions treated with rotational atherectomy and directional coronary atherectomy than in those treated with rotational atherectomy and adjunct balloon angioplasty.*

Ellis SG, Popma JJ, Buchbinder M, et al. Relation of clinical presentation, stenosis morphology, and operator technique to the procedural results of rotational atherectomy and rotational atherectomy-facilitated angioplasty. Circ. 1994;89(2):882–92. *Analysis of 400 lesions 316 patients randomly selected from the initial RA experience at 3 institutions showed 24% Type A, 40% Type B1, 30% Type B2 and 6% Type C lesions. Eighty-two percent had adjunctive PTCA with procedural success in 89.8% (93.5% if CPK 2–3x normal is not counted). Complications of no flow 3.8% and slow flow 5.1% correlated with burr time, right coronary stenosis and recent MI. Procedure failure correlated to no flow, lesion irregularity, angulation > 60, and female sex. Complications were death 0.3%, non-Qwave MI 5.7%, Qwave MI 2.2% and CABG 0.9% and occurred in 8.9% of patients.*

Erbel R, O'Neill WW, Auth D, et al. High-frequency rotational atherectomy in coronary heart disease. [German] Deutsche Medizinische Wochenschrift 1989; 114(13):487–95. *This is an early report of RA in 10 patients.*

Farb A, Roberts DK, Pichard AD, et al. Coronary artery morphologic features after coronary rotational atherectomy: Insights into mechanisms of lumen enlargement and embolization. Amer Heart J 1995; 129(6):1,058–67. *Autopsy was performed on two patients who died post-RA and balloon angioplasty. The luminal surfaces of the arteries were relatively smooth with focal unevenness where there was extensive nodular calcium. Atheroemboli were present where there was extensive nodular Ca but only one embolus was found with moderate Ca. There were numerous plaque fissures and a medial dissection which may have been secondary to the post RA balloon.*

Fourrier JL, Bertrand ME, Auth DC, et al. Percutaneous Coronary Rotational Angioplasty in Humans: Preliminary Report. J Amer Coll Cardiol, 1989; 14:1,278–82.

Gilmore PS, Bass TA, Conetta DA, et al. Single site experience with high-speed coronary rotational atherectomy. Clinical Cardiol 1993; 16(4): 311–6. *Single site experience with 108 patients, 143 lesions showed success in 99/108 patients and 131/143 lesions. Complications included 1 death, 1 Qwave MI, 3 non-Qwave MI and 3 CABGs. No patient related variables including age, gender, diabetes, hypertension, cigarette use, restenosis, previous MI or left ventricular function were predictive of poor outcome. No lesion characteristics were predictive of poor outcome.*

Guerin Y, Rahal S, Desnos M, et al. Coronary angioplasty combining rotational atherectomy and balloon dilatation. Results in 67 complex stenoses. [Italian] Archives des Maladies du Coeur et des Vaisseaux 1993; 86(11):1,535–41. *This is a study of RA followed by PTCA in type B2 lesions in 61 patients, 67 lesions. Treatment with a medium sized burr (50–70% reference diameter) was followed by the lowest balloon pressure possible for dilatation. Treatment success was achieved in 57 patients (93.4%). The mean balloon inflation pressure was 4.1 ATM There was (1) CABG, (1) Qwave MI and (2) technical failures. During atherectomy transient conduction defects occurred in 6.6%, severe hypotension in 3.3% and complete spasm in 4.5%.*

Guzman LA, Simpfendorfer C, Fix J, et al. Comparison of costs of new atherectomy devices and balloon angioplasty for coronary artery disease. Amer J Cardiol 1994; 74(1):22–5. *A comparison of the costs of PTCA with atherectomy using 65 DCA, 44 RA and 17 extraction with 126 PTCA patients matched for age and sex. The number of devices/procedure was 1.3 ± 0.6 for PTCA and 2.4 ± 1 for atherectomy. There were no differences in cost of hospital stay, procedure room, pharmacy or laboratory but supply cost was higher for the atherectomy group ($2,028 vs. $3,632). The mean cost of angioplasty was $7,301 ± 4,637 and of atherectomy was $9,345 ± 8,856. Clinical and procedural outcomes were similar.*

Hansen DD, Auth DC, Vracko R, et al. Rotational thrombectomy in acute canine coronary thrombosis. Internat J Cardiol. 1988; 22:13–19.

Hansen DD, Auth DC, Vracko R, et al. Mechanical thrombectomy: A comparison of two rotational devices and balloon angioplasty in subacute canine femoral thrombosis. Amer Heart. 1987;1:223–31.

Hansen DD, Intlekofer MJ, Hall M, et al. In-vivo rotational endarterectomy in canine coronary arteries. Lasers in Surgery Medicine, 1987;7:82-5.

Hansen DD, Auth DC, Vracko R, et al. Rotational atherectomy in atherosclerotic rabbit iliac arteries. Amer Heart J 1988; 115(1 Pt 1):160–5. *RA was tested in rabbit iliac arteries with atherosclerotic disease induced. Stenosis was decreased from 81% to 38% by RA. Histological examination revealed a smooth interior with intima removed. Particle collection resulted in 98% of particles < 10 microns is size.*

Henson KD, Popma JJ, Leon MB, et al. Comparison of results of rotational coronary atherectomy in three age groups (< 70, 70 to 79 and > or = 80 years). Amer J Cardiol 1993; 71(10):862–4. *A* *total of 412 patients were compared, 269 < 70 years, 119 were 70–79 and 24 > 80 years. Men were fewer in the oldest age group but other demographic variables were similar including ejection fraction. Lesions were calcified (76%), eccentric (73%), angulated (29%) and ostial (22%). Adjunctive PTCA was used in 82% with a final residual stenosis of 26% post-procedure. Procedural success was 95% and tended to be lower 87.5% in the very elderly. At 1 year follow-up freedom from major clinical events was obtained in 84% pts < 70, 87% pts 70–79 and 71% pts > 80. Within 6 months 17% of patients < 70 had repeat revascularization while 6% of those > 70 had repeat procedures.*

Hong MK, Mintz GS, Popma JJ, et al. Safety and efficacy of elective stent implantation following rotational atherectomy in large calcified coronary arteries. Cathet Cardiovasc Diag 1996; Supple 3:50–54. *Twenty-four patients were treated by rotational atherectomy followed by implantation of coronary artery stents. The lesions were heavily calcified. Procedural success was 100% with no acute complications and no sub acute thrombosis in 30 days.*

Khoury A, Kern M, Coronary physiology of percutaneous rotational atherectomy. Cathet Cardiovasc Diag 1996; Supple 3:15–22. *A review of Doppler flow velocity measurements before and after rotational atherectomy which suggests that coronary flow reserve may not improve post-atherectomy despite significant angiographic improvements.*

Khoury AF, Aguirre FV, Bach RG, et al. Influence of percutaneous transluminal coronary rotational atherectomy with adjunctive percutaneous transluminal coronary angioplasty on coronary blood flow. Amer Heart J. 1996; 131(4):631–8. *PTCRA in 14 lesions significantly increased resting coronary blood flow measured before and after RA and adjunctive angioplasty using a Doppler flow wire. Adjunctive balloon angioplasty did not significantly augment resting or hyperemic coronary blood flow more than that achieved by rotational atherectomy alone. These data demonstrate that PTCRA alone improves baseline coronary blood flow with minimal additional physiologic change after adjunctive balloon angioplasty.*

Khoury AF, Bach RG, Kern MJ, et al. Influence of adjunctive balloon angioplasty on coronary blood flow after rotational atherectomy Cathet Cardiovasc Diag. 1995; 36(3):272–6. *This case study reports the normalization of coronary flow reserve after angioplasty in a patient undergoing RA + angioplasty.*

Koller PT, Freed M, Grines CL, et al. Success, complications, and restenosis following rotational and transluminal extraction atherectomy of ostial stenoses. Cathet Cardiovasc Diag 1994; 31(4):255–60. *RA in 29 patients and DCA in 72 patients were performed on ostial lesions with high success (93% and 90%) and low complication (6.9% and 4.2%). Adjunctive balloon was required in 85% of patients. The restenosis rates were 39% and 66%. The higher restenosis in DCA was due to restenosis in vein grafts. There was no difference in restenosis rates in coronary arteries.*

Kovach JA, Mintz GS, Pichard AD, et al. Sequential intravascular ultrasound characterization of the mechanisms of rotational atherectomy and adjunct balloon angioplasty. J Amer Coll Cardiol 1993; 22(4):1,024–32. *Intravascular ultrasound was used to examine 46 lesions pre treatment, post-RA and in 44/46 post-PTCA. After RA lumen area increased, plaque plus media area decreased, target lesion calcium decreased and 26% of target lesions had dissection planes. After balloon angioplasty, external elastic membrane area increased, lumen area decreased, plaque plus media did not change and 77% of lesions had dissection planes. The pattern of dissection plane location was predominately within calcified plaque after RA and adjacent to calcified plaque after PTCA.*

Levin TN, Carroll J, Feldman T. High-speed rotational atherectomy of chronic total coronary occlusions. Cathet Cardiovasc Diag 1996; Supple 3:34–39. *This report summarizes the treatment of 15 chronic total occlusions with RA. The procedure was successful in all lesions with no major complications. In follow-up 2 patients had required revascularization, with no MIs or deaths.*

Lotan C, Rozenman Y, Weiss AT, et al. Urgent rotational ablation of a partially protected, totally occluded left main coronary artery. Cathet Cardiovasc Diag 1996; Supple 3:78–81. *A case report of rotational atherectomy of a left main stenosis in a patient whose left main bypass graft failed four months post surgery.*

MacIsaac AI, Bass TA, Buchbinder M, et al. High-speed rotational atherectomy: Outcome in calcified and noncalcified coronary artery lesions. J Amer Coll Cardiol 1995; 26(3):531–6. *The study compares the lesions and results from 2,161 procedures, 1,078 with calcified lesions and 1,083 noncalcified lesions. Patients with calcified lesions were older. The lesions were more frequently new, angulated, eccentric, and > 10 mm in length. They were more often complex and located in the LAD. Adjunctive PTCA was used in 83% of calcified and 67% of noncalcified lesions. Procedural success was 94.3% in calcified and 95.2% in noncalcified lesions with residual stenosis of 21.6% in calcified and 23.3% in noncalcified lesions. The rate of major complications was not different between the two groups. The rate of non Qwave MI was higher in the calcified group 10% vs. 7.7% P=0.05).*

Mintz GS, Douek P, Pichard AD, et al. Target lesion calcification in coronary artery disease: an intravascular ultrasound study. J Amer Coll Cardiol 1992; 20(5):1,149–55. *IVUS was performed in 110 patients. Eighty-four percent had target lesion calcification by IVUS, 29 in one quadrant, 25 in two quadrants, 17 in three and 13 in four. Calcium was superficial in 42, deep in 13 and both in 31 patients. The axial length of calcium measured in 29 patients was < 5 mm in 11 and > 6 in 18. Fluoroscopy detected Ca in 50 patients, in 74% of patients with 2 or more quadrants of calcium and in 86% of patients with Ca > 6 mm in two or more quadrants. Calcification was more common in patients who smoked and tended to be more common in people with multivessel disease.*

Mintz GS, Pichard AD, Kovach JA, et al. Impact of preintervention intravascular ultrasound imaging on transcatheter treatment strategies in coronary artery disease. Amer J Cardiol 1994;

73(7):423–30. *Strategy for treatment intended before IVUS and actual treatment were compared in 313 lesions 301 patients. There was a change in treatment in 124 lesions 121 patients (40%). Changes included revascularization due to more severe lesion (20, 6%), no revascularization due to less severe lesion (21, 7%), assessment of lesion composition leading to change in strategy (20, 6%) or change in reason for selecting device (63, 20%). IVUS diameter correlated well with angiography (r= 0.83). Lesions with Ca were referred to RA, eccentric lesions without Ca to DCA, dissections and aneurysms to stent, thrombus containing lesions to thrombolytic therapy and fibrotic vein grafts to PTCA or stent.*

Mintz GS, Potkin BN, Keren G, et al. Intravascular ultrasound evaluation of the effect of rotational atherectomy in obstructive atherosclerotic coronary artery disease. Circ 1992; 86(5):1,383–93. *IVUS was used to examine the lesions of 28 patients after RA or after adjunctive PTCA. 79% of lesions were calcified. After RA the lumen was unusually distinct and circular. The lumen was larger than the largest burr for both stand alone RA and adjunctive PTCA. In the 5 patients studied before and after RA, IVUS showed an increase in lumen size, a decrease in plaque plus media and in target calcium and no change in external elastic membrane cross-sectional area.*

Mintz, GS, Pichard AD, Popma JJ, et al. Preliminary experience with adjunct directional coronary atherectomy after high-speed rotational atherectomy in the treatment of calcific coronary artery disease. Amer J Cardiol, 1993; 71(10):799–804. *RA followed by DCA was performed in 10 patients with calcified target lesions. Stenosis decreased from 78% to 50% after RA and to 17% after subsequent DCA.*

Murphy MC, Hansell HN, Ward K, et al. Differences in symptoms during and post-PTCA versus rotational ablation. Progress in Cardiovasc Nurs 1994; 9(2):4–9. *The study compared factors that would impact nursing in 233 patients undergoing RA with*

301 patients undergoing PTCA. RA patients were more likely to experience hypotension or prolonged angina in the cath lab and experienced longer post procedure heparin and NTG therapy. There was no difference in peripheral bleeding, hematoma or length of stay.

Nunez BD, Keelan ET, Higano ST, et al. Coronary hemodynamics before and after rotational atherectomy with adjunctive balloon angioplasty. Cathet Cardiovasc Diag 1996; Supple 3:40–49. *The Doppler Flow Wire was used to measure flow after atherectomy in 10 patients, 4 with normal flow and 6 with slow or no flow. Although flow returned to normal with vasodilators and balloon angioplasty, coronary flow reserve did not increase post-procedure.*

O'Murchu B, Foreman RD, Shaw RE, et al. Role of the intra-aortic balloon pump counterpulsation in high risk coronary atherectomy. J Amer Coll Cardiol 1995; 26 (5):1,270–5. *The study compared the outcomes of 28 high risk patients in whom a balloon pump was placed electively before the procedure to 131 high risk patients 5 of whom required a balloon pump emergently during the procedure. Slow flow occurred in 18% of each group. Among patients with slow flow, non-Qwave infarction occurred only in the second group and elective balloon placement was the only variable to correlate with a successful procedure uncomplicated by hypotension.*

Pavlides GS, Hauser AM, Grines CL, et al. Clinical, hemodynamic, electrocardiographic and mechanical events during nonocclusive, coronary atherectomy and comparison with balloon angioplasty. Amer J Cardiol. 1992; 70(9):841–5. *A comparison of the events surrounding RA (17 patients), TEC (18 patients) were compared with the events during PTCA of the 16/17 and 14/18 patients who underwent adjunctive PTCA. Chest pain was more frequent during PTCA while ST changes were similar in all three. 6 patients had transient AV block during RA compared with none during TEC or PTCA. Hemodynamic parameters and left ventricular function were not affected by atherectomy. Wall motion score in the region of the target artery was not affected during RA but was decreased slightly during TEC and more during PTCA (0.3 to 1.0 to 2.0 respectively).*

Popma JJ, Brogan WCD, Pichard A, et al. Rotational coronary atherectomy of ostial stenoses. Amer J of Cardiol 1993; 71(5):436–8. *Treatment of 105 patients with ostial lesions by RA followed by PTCA in 85% is reported. RA reduced stenosis from 73% to 41% and PTCA further reduced it to 23%. Success was obtained in 97% of lesions. Dissections developed in 18 patients, 7 were minor, spasm occurred in 3 patients and responded to dilators and balloon, 2 patients received CABG. There were no deaths. During follow-up 34% of patients developed recurrent angina and angiographic restenosis was present in 23/73 (32%) of patients. Four patients died in follow-up.*

Razzolini R, Chioin. Rotational atherectomy and PTCA in complex coronary lesions (B2 and C): the immediate and long-term results. [Italian] Giornale Italiano di Cardiologia. 1995; 25(9):1,127–38. *This study reports on 26 type B2 and C lesions treated with RA. Procedural success was achieved in 92% with angina or a positive stress test found in 45% on follow-up.*

Reisman M. Technique and strategy of rotational atherectomy. Cathet Cardiovasc Diag 1996; Supple 3:2–14. *A review of new advances in the application of rotational atherectomy.*

Reisman M, Harms V. Guidewire bias: A potential source of complications with rotational atherectomy. Cathet Cardiovasc Diag 1996; Supple 3:64–8. *An analysis of the role of guidewire bias in contributing to complications using three case studies as examples.*

Reisman M, Buchbinder M. Rotational ablation. The Rotablator catheter. Cardiol Clinics 1994 12(4):595–610. *This article summarizes results, identifies indications and discusses potential applications of RA in the treatment of coronary artery disease.*

Rosenblum J., O'Donnell MJ, Sterzer SH, et al. Rotational ablation of a severely angulated stenosis previously not amenable to balloon angioplasty. Amer Heart J 1991; 122(6):1,766–8.

Rosenblum J, Stertzer SH, Schechtmann NS, et al. Brachial rotational atherectomy. Cathet Cardiovasc Diag 1991; 24(1): 32–6. *A case study of two cases of RA using a brachial approach.*

Rozenman Y, Lotan C, Weiss AT, et al. Emergency rotational ablation of a calcified left main coronary artery stenosis in a patient with ischemic induced cardiogenic shock. Cathet Cardiovasc Diag. 1995; 36(1):63–6. *This report describes the treatment of a left main stenosis in an elderly woman in cardiogenic shock secondary to vein graft failure.*

Ruygrok PN., Pasteuning WH., de Jaegere PP., et al. Angina after successful coronary atherectomy. Amer Heart J. 1995;130(6):1309–11

Sabri MN, Cowley MJ, DiSciascio G, et al. Immediate results of interventional devices for coronary ostial narrowing with angina pectoris. Amer J Cardiol 1994; 73(2): 122–5. *Thirty-one lesions in 29 patients having ostial lesions were treated with a new device (DCA 8, RA 4, Laser 17) followed by PTCA and compared to a group of 15 patient receiving PTCA alone. Percent reduction in stenosis was 66% DCA, 67% RA, 52% laser and 46% PTCA. Procedural success was 91% with new devices and 93% with PTCA alone.*

Safian RD, Freed M, Lichtenberg A, et al. Are residual stenoses after excimer laser angioplasty and coronary atherectomy due to inefficient or small devices? Comparison with balloon angioplasty. J Amer Coll Cardiol 1993; 22(6): 1,628–34. *The study compared minimum luminal diameter and percent diameter stenosis in 696 patients treated with either RA, extraction atherectomy, to PTCA. The percent diameter stenosis was greater post new device compared to balloon. The ratio of device diameter to artery size was smaller for the new devices than for balloon. The ratio of device diameter to post device artery diameter was highest for RA 0.92 ± 0.16 indicating an efficient device with little immediate recoil.*

Safian RD, Niazi KA, Strzelecki M, et al. Detailed angiographic analysis of high-speed mechanical rotational atherectomy in human coronary arteries. Circ 1993; 88(3): 961–8. *Angiographic examination of 116 lesions from 104 patients treated with RA (23%) or RA + PTCA (77%) showed a decrease in stenosis to 70 ± 13% to 54 ± 23% post RA to 30 ± 20% post procedure. The minimum luminal diameter increased from 1.0 ± 0.5 mm to 1.4 ± 0.7 post-RA to 2.3 ± 0.7 post-procedure. The minimum luminal diameter post RA was 91% of burr diameter. Significant complications included abrupt closure 11%, no reflow 7%, severe spasm 14% and guidewire fracture 3%. Clinical complications included Qwave MI 5%, non-Qwave MI 3%, femoral vascular injury requiring surgery 3%, transfusion 8%, CABG 2% and death 1%. Angiographic follow-up in 84% of patients revealed restenosis rate of 51%.*

Safian RD, Freed M, Lichtenberg A, et al. Usefulness of percutaneous transluminal coronary angioplasty after new device coronary interventions. Amer J Cardiol 1994;73(9): 642–6. *PTCA was used after 83% of new device interventions (85% of 290 extraction, 72% of 79 RA and 89% of 118 laser) Device success was defined as > 20% reduction in stenosis and procedural success as < 50% final stenosis, salvage PTCA was defined as PTCA to manage device induced occlusion. PTCA was used to enlarge the lumen after device success in only 28.5% of cases and was used for minimal or no change in diameter in 50% and worsening diameter in 21.5%. Salvage PTCA was performed in 12.6% of lesions. Procedural success was 85% with a low incidence of complications.*

Safian RD, Freed M, Reddy V, et al. Do excimer laser angioplasty and rotational atherectomy facilitate balloon angioplasty? Implications for lesion-specific coronary intervention. J Amer

Coll Cardiol. 1996; 27(3):552–9. *This study compared the final luminal diameter and the final diameter to balloon ratio in lesions treated with balloon alone (n = 541), extraction atherectomy + balloon (n = 277), rotational atherectomy + balloon (n = 211) or excimer laser + balloon (n = 237). Final residual stenosis was smaller with RA and the efficiency of the balloon was greater with RA for ostial, eccentric, calcified or long lesions.*

Schechtmann N, Rosenblum J, Stertzer S, et al. Rotational ablation of chronic coronary occlusions, Cathet Cardiovasc Diag, 1991;24:295–299.

Schofer J, Geiger B, Kunze KP, et al. [Does rotablation of complex coronary artery stenosis lower the risk of subsequent PTCA?] (German) Z Kardiol 1994; 83(1): 24–30. *RA before angioplasty in complex lesions (Type B &C) improved success from 83% of 250 to 87% of 437 with 102 treated with RA first. Dissection rate was similar but those in second group (119 RA + balloon 318 balloon only) were more easily controlled and had a lower rate of major complication due to dissection (2.5 vs. 4.4)*

Sievert H, Tonndorf S, Utech A, et al. [High frequency rotational angioplasty (rotablation) after unsuccessful balloon dilatation]. (German) Z Kardiol 1993; 82(7: 411–4). *In 36/2,442 patients scheduled for angioplasty a guidewire could be passed but not the balloon. In 32/36 cases the Type C guidewire was exchanged and 15 cases were treated with RA alone while 17 were treated with RA + PTCA. A stent was required in one patient. Stenosis went from 95 ± 10% to 33 ± 6%.*

Stertzer SH, Pomerantsev EV, Shaw RE, et al. Comparative study of the angiographic morphology of coronary artery lesions treated with PTCA, directional coronary atherectomy, or high-speed rotational ablation. Cathet Cardiovasc Diag 1994; 33(1): 1–9. *Morphology of lesions (110 lesions each) treated with PTCA, DCA or RA were compared. PTCA was used mainly in discrete, concentric, smooth, ACC/AHA type A and B1 lesions. It was used less frequently on a bend, branch point or calcified lesions. DCA was used in discrete, proximal, eccentric and noncalcified lesions. RA was used in diffuse, calcified, multiple complicated type B2 and C lesions with sidebranches and bend points. Success and complication rates were similar for all three.*

Stertzer SH, Rosenblum J, Shaw RE, et al. Coronary rotational ablation: initial experience in 302 procedures. J Amer Coll Cardiol 1993; 21(2): 287–95. *A series of 242 patients having 302 procedures involving 308 vessels and 346 lesions were treated with RA. Of the 346 lesions 320 (92.5%) were type B or C. 119 patients had had previous PTCA attempts, 31 had been unsuccessful. Left ventricular ejection fraction was normal for 81%. Procedural success was achieved for 284/302 (94%) procedures and 330/346 (95.4%) lesions. A major cardiac event occurred in 13 cases. Follow-up of 182 patients showed 95.4% alive and free of MI. Angiographic follow-up was available in 87 patients. Estimated restenosis from clinical and angiographic follow-up was 37.4%.*

Stertzer SH, Pomerantsev EV, Fitzgerald PJ, et al. High-speed rotational atherectomy: Six-month serial quantitative coronary angiographic follow-up. Amer Heart J 1996; 131(4):639–48. *Angiography of 123 patients 7 months after RA showed that the restenotic lesions were more focal and less complex than the original lesion. More complex baseline lesions were in the group with highest net gain at six months, the group with the highest initial gain and lowest late loss. The restenosis rate in this group was 6%.*

Stertzer S, Rosenblum J, Shaw, R, et al. Restenosis following successful rotational ablation of de novo coronary stenosis. J Invas Cardiol, 1993;5:295–302.

Stone GW. Rotational atherectomy for treatment of in-stent restenosis: Role of intracoronary ultrasound guidance. Cathet Cardiovasc Diag 1996; Supple 3:73–77. *A case report of rotational atherectomy to treat in-stent restenosis.*

Tamburino C, Corcos T, Favereau X, et al. [Preliminary experience in the treatment of complex stenosis in the aged (> or = 70 years) with high-speed rotational atherectomy followed by conventional PTCA]. (Italian) Giornale Italiano di Cardiologia 1994; 24(6): 701–5. *Complex lesions (n=46) in 36 patients over the age of 70 were treated with RA and angioplasty. The procedure was successful in 94% of patients, 2 patients had major complications (1 CABG and one MI). No patient showed significant deterioration of residual stenosis at 24 hours. Lesion characteristics were eccentric 63%, calcified 69%, angulated 44%, longer than 10 mm 11%, undilatable 11%, ostial 9% and ulcerated 7%.*

Teirstein PS, Warth DC, Hag N, et al. High-speed rotational coronary atherectomy for patients with diffuse coronary artery disease J Amer Coll Cardiol 1991; 18(7): 1694–701. *Forty-two patients 71% with lesions > 10 mm were treated with RA alone. Overall procedural success was 76%, 92% in lesions < 10 mm and 70% in lesion > 10 mm. Complications included 1 CABG who subsequently died, 8 non-Qwave MI which correlated with lesion length. 4/8 of these patients had transient left ventricular wall motion abnormalities. Follow-up angiography in 91% showed restenosis of 59%, 22% in lesions< 10 mm and 75% in lesions >10 mm.*

Titus B, Auth D, Ritchie J. Distal embolization during mechanical thrombolysis: rotational thrombectomy vs. balloon angioplasty, Cathet Cardiovasc Diag, 1990;19:279–285.

Tsocanakis O, Guerin F, Guerot C. Rotational atherectomy with adjunctive balloon angioplasty versus conventional percutaneous transluminal coronary angioplasty in type B2 lesions: results of a randomized study. Amer Heart J. 1996; 131(5):879–83. *This study randomized 64 patients with Type B2 lesions to primary angioplasty or RA using a single medium sized burr with adjunctive angioplasty. In this small series there were no differences in procedural success or angiographic restenosis in the two groups.*

van de Rijn M, Regula Jr. DP, et al. Autopsy findings after coronary rotational atherectomy. Amer J Cardiovasc Path 1990; 3(4):301–4. *This is an autopsy report of a single patient who after RA developed abrupt closure and was treated with balloon and CABG and died two days later of cardiac failure. There was no evidence of perforation or dissection. Thrombus was present and downstream of the treated artery small arteries and arterioles were embolized by pulverized atheroma.*

von Birgelen C, Umans VA, Di Mario C, et al. Mechanism of high-speed rotational atherectomy and adjunctive balloon angioplasty revisited by quantitative coronary angiography: edge detection versus videodensitometry. Amer Heart J. 1995; 130(3 Pt 1):405–12. *This study compares edge detection to videodensitometry for QCA in 21 lesions. Edge detection and videodensitometry provided equivalent immediate angiographic results after RA and adjunctive BA.*

Waksman R, King SBR, Douglas JS, et al. Predictors of groin complications after balloon and new-device coronary intervention. Amer J Cardiol 1995; 75(14): 886–9. *Vascular complications occurred in 309/5,042 patients, 117 (2.3%) of whom required surgical repair. Correlates of repair were increased age, female gender, increased weight, higher systolic blood pressure, increased heparin during procedure, receiving heparin post procedure and stenting. Sheath size and device other than stent did not correlate with vascular complication.*

Walton AS, Pomerantsev EV, Oesterle SN, et al. Outcome of narrowing related side branches after high-speed rotational atherectomy. Amer J Cardiol. 1996; 77(5):370–3. *This study was performed to determine the rate, predictors, and outcome of side branch occlusion after RA. Angiograms of 418 patients revealed 320 side branches > 1 mm in 240 target vessels. Post-procedure they were occluded in 21 patients. Angiography at 24 hours showed 12/13 to be patent. In the 21 patients with occluded vessels, 6 sustained MIs, 2 underwent bypass and 2 died.*

Warth DC, Leon MB, O'Neill W, et al. Rotational atherectomy multicenter registry: Acute results, complications and 6-month angiographic follow-up in 709 patients. J Amer Coll Cardiol 1994; 24(3): 641–8. *A report of the registry in 709 patients, 743 procedures and 874 lesions. Lesions were eccentric 61%, calcified 31% tortuous 27%, and long 25%. Procedural success was 94.7% and did not vary with lesion type location or severity. Previously treated lesions had a higher success rate 97.4%. Major complication occurred at rates of death 0.8%, Qwave MI 0.9% and CABG 1.7% and were associated with length and number of lesions treated. Non-Qwave MI occurred in 3.8% and was associated with females and history of MI. Abrupt occlusion occurred in 3.1% and was associated with bifurcated lesions and adjunctive therapy. Dissection was seen in 10.5% and was associated with more complex lesions. Restenosis rate was 37.7% at 6 months (done in 64% of patients). Restenosis was associated with poorer initial treatment outcome and diabetes.*

Zacca NM, Kleiman NS, Rodriguez AR, et al. Rotational ablation of coronary artery lesions using single, large burrs. Cathet Cardiovasc Diag 1992; 26(2): 92–7. *This study tested the efficacy of a single large burr (>2.25 mm, 70–90% luminal diameter) without adjunctive angioplasty in 31 patients with 36 complex lesions. Diameter stenosis was reduced from 69.8 ± 11.3% to 30.9 ± 10%. There were 4 dissections, 2 uncomplicated. A third patient had a Qwave MI and a fourth had abrupt closure 36 hours later and underwent CABG.*

Zimarino M, Corcos T, Favereau X, et al. Rotational coronary atherectomy with adjunctive balloon angioplasty for the treatment of ostial lesions. Cathet Cardiovasc Diag 1994; 33(1): 22–7. *Ostial lesions (OL) were treated by RA followed by PTCA in 63 patients (69 lesions). Procedural success was achieved in 58 patients (92%) with success in 14/15 aorto-OL (93%) and 50/54 branch-OL (93%). Major complications occurred in 2 patients and uncomplicated failure occurred in 3 patients. Diameter stenosis decreased from 75 ± 13% preprocedure to 32 ± 12 post RA to 14 ± 10% post-PTCA. At 24 hour repeat angiography diameter stenosis was 17 ± 15% with no patient >50%. Follow-up angiography was performed in 30 patients who had an abnormal stress test: 13 of 30 showed angiographic restenosis of at least one successfully treated OL.*

Zotz R, Stahr P, Erbel R, et al. Analysis of high-frequency rotational angioplasty-induced echo contrast. Cathet Cardiovasc Diag, 1991;22:137–144.

Zotz, R, Erbel R, Philipp A, et al. High-speed rotational angioplasty-induced echo contrast in vivo and in vitro optical analysis. Cathet Cardiovasc Diag, 1992;26:98–110.

References

1. Hansen DD, Auth DC, Vracko R, et. al. Rotational atherectomy in atherosclerotic rabbit iliac arteries. Am Heart J 1988; 115:160–165.

2. Ahn SS, Auth DC, Marcus DR, et al. Removal of focal atheromatous lesions by angioscopically guided high-speed rotary atherectomy: Preliminary experimental observations. J Vasc Surg 1988; 7:292–300.

3. Hansen DH, Auth DC, Hall M, et.al. Rotational endarterectomy in normal canine coronary arteries: preliminary report. J Am Coll Cardiol 1988; 11:1073–77.

4. Fourrier JL, Bertrand ME, Auth DC, et al. Percutaneous coronary rotational angioplasty in humans: preliminary report. J Am Coll Cardiol 1989; 14:1278–82.

5. Mintz GS, Potkin BN, Keren G, et al. Intravascular ultrasound evaluation of the effect of rotational atherectomy in obstructive atherosclerotic coronary artery disease. Circulation 1992; 86(5):1383–93.

6. Potkin BN, Mintz GS, Matar FA, et al. A mechanistic comparison of transcatheter therapies assessed by intravascular ultrasound (abstract). Circulation 1991; 84:II–541.

7. Kovach JA, Mintz GS, Pichard AD, et al. Sequential intravascular ultrasound characterization of the mechanisms of rotational atherectomy and adjunct balloon angioplasty. J Am Coll Cardiol 1993; 22(4):1024–32.

8. Cowley M, Buchbinder M, Warth D, et al. Effect of coronary rotational atherectomy abrasion on vessel segments adjacent to treated lesions (abstract). J Am Coll Cardiol 1992; 19:333A.

9. Prevosti LG, Cook JA, Unger EF, et al. Particulate debris from rotational atherectomy: size distribution and physiologic effects (abstract). Circulation 1988; 78:II–83.

10. Friedman HZ, Elliot MA, Gottlieb GJ, et al. Mechanical rotary atherectomy: The effects of microparticle embolization on myocardial blood flow and function. J Int Cardiol 1989; 2:77–83.

11. Sherman CT, Brunken R, Chan A, et al. Myocardial perfusion and segmental wall motion after coronary rotational atherectomy (abstract). Circulation 1992; 86:I–652.

12. Pavlides GS, Hauser AM, Grines CL, et al. Clinical, hemodynamic, electrocardiographic and mechanical events during non-occlusive coronary atherectomy and comparison with balloon angioplasty. Am J Cardiol 1992 70:841–845.

13. Huggins GS, Williams MJA, Yang J, et al. Transient wall motion abnormalities following rotational atherectomy are reflective of myocardial stunning more than myocardial infarction (abstract). J Am Coll Cardiol 1995; 25:96A.

14. Williams MJA, Dow CJ, Weyman AE, et al. Myocardial dysfunction after rotational coronary atherectomy: Serial evaluation by echocardiography (abstract). Circulation.1994; 90 (4): I-395.

15. Zotz RJ, Erbel R, Phillip A, et al. High-speed rotational angioplasty-induced echo contrast in vivo and in vitro optical analysis. Cathet Cardiovasc Diagn 1992; 26:98–109.

16. Reisman M, Buchbinder M, Bass T, et al. Improvement in coronary dimensions at early 24-hour follow-up after coronary rotational ablation: Implications for restenosis (abstract). Circulation 1992; 86:I–332.

17. Safian RD, Freed M, Lictenberg A, et al: Are residual stenoses after excimer laser angioplasty and coronary atherectomy due to inefficient or small devices? J Am Coll Cardiol 1993; 22:1628–34.

18. Mintz GS, Potkin BN, Keren G, et al. Cross-sectional and three-dimensional intravascular ultrasound analysis of coronary artery geometry after rotational atherectomy [abstract]. Circulation 1994;90:I–203.

19. Hong MK, Tjurmin A, Haudenschild CC, et al. Historical finding in directional atherectomy specimens after rotational atherectomy in calcified coronary arteries (abstract). Circulation 1994; 90:I–213.

20. Reisman M, DeVore LJ, Ferguson M, et al. Anaysis of heat generation during high-speed rotational ablation: Technical implication (abstract). J Am Coll Cardiol 1996; 27:292A.

21. Reisman M, Shuman B, Fei R, et al. Analysis and comparison of platelet aggregation with high-speed rotational atherectomy (abstract) J Am Coll Cardiol 1997;27:186A

22. Yamashita K, Satake S, Ottira H, et al. Radiofrequency thermal balloon coronary angioplasty: a new device for successful percutaneous transluminal coronary angioplasty. J Am Coll Cardiol 1994; February 23(2):336–40.

23. Reis GJ, Pomerantz M, et al. Laser balloon angioplasty: clinical, angiographic and histological results. J Am Coll Cardiol 1991; 8:193–202.

24 Snabre P, Baumler H, Mills P, et al. Aggregation of human red blood cells after moderate heat treatment. Biorheology 1985; 22: 185–195.

25. Lapshina EA, Biokizika IB, Thermal stability of erythrocyte membrane proteins at varying ionic strength and media composition. Biofizika 1994; Nov–Dec 396(6):1015–20.

26. Gader AM, Mashhadani, Direct activation of platelets by heat is the possible trigger of the coagulopathy of heat stroke. Br. J. Haematol 1990; January 74(1):86–92.

27. Warth DC, Leon MB, O'Neill W, et al. Rotational atherectomy multicenter registry: acute results, complications and 6-month angiographic follow-up in 709 patients. J Am Coll Cardiol 1994; 24(3):641–8.

28. Stertzer SH, Rosenblum J, Shaw RE, et al. Coronary rotational ablation: Initial experience in 302 procedures [see comments]. J Am Coll Cardiol 1993; 21(2):287–95.

29. Safian RD, Niazi KA, Strzelecki M, et al. Detailed angiographic analysis of high-speed mechanical rotational atherectomy in human coronary arteries. Circulation 1993; 88(3):961–8.

30. Teirstein PS, Warth DC, Haq N, et al: High-speed rotational coronary atherectomy for patients with diffuse coronary artery disease. J Am Coll Cardiol 1991; 18:1,694–1,701.

31. Borrione M, Hall P, Almagor Y, et al. Treatment of simple and complex coronary stenosis using rotational ablation followed by low-pressure balloon angioplasty. Cathet. Cardiovasc Diagn 1993; 30(2):131–7.

32. Gilmore PS, Bass TA, Conetta DA, et al.Single site experience with high-speed coronary rotational atherectomy. Clin. Cardiol. 1993; 16(4):311–6.

33. Guerin Y, Rahal S, Desnos M, et al. [Coronary angioplasty combining rotational atherectomy and balloon dilatation. Results in 67 complex stenoses]. Arch. des Maladies du Coeur et des Vaisseaux 1993; 86(11):1,535–41.

34. Dietz U, Erbel R, Rupprecht HJ, et al. High frequency rotational ablation: An alternative in treating coronary artery stenoses and occlusions. British Heart J 1993; 70(4):327–36.

35. Ellis SG, Popma JJ, Buchbinder M, et al. Relation of clinical presentation, stenosis morphology, and operator technique to the procedural results of rotational atherectomy and rotational atherectomy-facilitated angioplasty. Circulation 1994; 89(2):882–92.

36. Vandormael M, Reifart N, Preusler W, et al. Comparison of excimer laser, rotablator and balloon angioplasty for the treatment of complex lesions: ERBAC study final results

(abstract). J Am Coll Cardiol 1994; 23(2):57A.

37. MacIsaac AI, Bass TA, Buchbinder M, et al. High-speed rotational atherectomy: Outcome in calcified and noncalcified coronary artery lesions. J Am Coll Cardiol 1995; 26(3):531–6.

38. Altmann D, Popma J, Kent K, et al. Rotational atherectomy effectively treats calcified lesions (abstract). J Am Coll Cardiol 1993; 21(2):955A.

39. Reisman M, Cohen B, Warth D, et al. Outcome of long lesions treated with high–speed rotational ablation (abstract). J Am Coll Cardiol 1993; 21(2):443A.

40. Favereau X, Chevalier B, Commeau P, et al. Is rotational atherectomy more effective than balloon angioplasty for the treatment of long coronary lesions? (abstract) J Invas Cardiol 1994; 4:3A.

41. Koller PT, Freed M, Grines CL, et al. Success, complications, and restenosis following rotational and transluminal extraction atherectomy of ostial stenoses. Cathet Cardiovasc Diagn 1994; 31:255–60.

42. Popma J, Brogan W, Pichard A, et al. Rotational coronary atherectomy of ostial stenoses. Am J Cardiol 1993; 71(5): 436–8.

43. Zimarino M, Corcos T, Favereau X, et al. Rotational coronary atherectomy with adjunctive balloon angioplasty for the treatment of ostial lesions. Cathet Cardiovasc Diagn 1994; 33:22–7.

44. Omoigui N, Booth J, Reisman M, et al. Rotational atherectomy in chronic total occlusions (abstract). J Am Coll Cardiol 1995; 25:97A.

45. Reisman M, Devlin P, Melikian J, et al. Undilatable noncompliant lesions treated with the Rotablator: outcome and angiographic follow-up (abstract). Circulation 1993; 88: I–547.

46. Brogan W, Popma J, Pichard A, et al. Rotational coronary atherectomy after unsuccessful coronary balloon angioplasty. Am J Cardiol 1993; 71(10):794–8.

47. Rosenblum J, Stertzer S, Shaw R, et al . Rotational ablation of balloon angioplasty failures. J Invas Cardiol 1992; 4(6): 312–7.

48. Sievert H, Tonndorf S, Utech A, et al. [High-frequency rotational angioplasty (rotablation) after unsuccessful balloon dilatation]. Z Cardiol. 1993; 82(7):411–4.

49. Bass T, Gilmore P, Buchbinder M, et al. Coronary rotational atherectomy (PTCRA) in patients with prior coronary revascularization: A registry report (abstract). Circulation 1992; 86 (4):I-653.

50. Chevalier B, Commeau P, Favereau X, et al. Limitations of rotational atherectomy in angulated coronary lesions (abstract). J Am Coll Cardiol 1994; 23:285A.

51. Kaplan BM, Mojoares JJ, Safian Rd, et al. Optimal burr and adjunctive balloon sizing alters the need for target vessel revascularization after rotational atherectomy (abstract). J Am Coll Cardiol 1996;27:291A.

52. Whitlow PL, Cowley MJ, Kuntz RE, et al. Study to determine Rotablator and transluminal angioplasty strategy (STRATAS): Acute results (abstract). Circulation 1996;94:I-435.

53. Eccleston DS, Horrigan MC, Cowley MJ, et al. Is there a role for strip chart recording to guide rotational atherectomy? Initial findings from STRATAS. (abstract) J Am Coll Cardiol 1996; 27(2):292A.

54. Horrigan MC, Eccleston DS, Williams DO, et al. Technique dependence of CKMB elevation after rotational atherectomy (abstract). Circulation 1996; 94:I-560.

55. Buchbinder MA, Braden GA, Sharma SK, et al. A pilot study of ReoPro with rotational atherectomy (RA) to reduce creatine kinase (CK) elevation post-procedure (abstract). Circulation 1996; 94:I-197.

56. Braden GA, Applegate RJ, Young TM, et al. ReoPro decreases creatine kinase elevation following rotational atherectomy: Evidence for a platelet dependent mechanism (abstract). Circulation 1996; 94:I-248.

57. Hong MK, Mintz GS, Popma JJ, et al. Safety and efficacy of elective stent implantation following rotational atherectomy

in large, calcified coronary arteries. Cathet Cardiovasc Diagn 1996; Suppl 3:50–4.

58. Mintz GS, Dussaillant GR, Wong SC, et al. Rotational atherectomy followed by adjunct stents: The preferred therapy for calcified large vessels? (abstract). Circulation 1995; 92:I–329.

59. Buchbinder MA, Goldberg SL, Fortuna R, et al. Rotational atherectomy for intra-stent restenosis: Initial experience (abstract). Circulation 1996; 94:I–621.

60. Reisman M, Buchbinder M, Warth D, et al. Comparison of patients with either < 70% diameter narrowing or > 70% narrowing of the right coronary artery when performing rotational rotational atherectomy on > 1 narrowing in the left coronary arteries. Am J Cardiol 1997; 79:305–8.

61. O'Murchu B, Foreman RD, Shaw RE, et al. Role of the intra-aortic balloon pump counterpulsation in high-risk coronary atherectomy. J Am Coll Cardiol 1995; 26(5):1270–5.

62. Cohen BM, Weber VJ, Blum RR, et al. Cocktail attenuation of rotational ablation flow effects (CARAFE) study: Pilot. Cathet Cardiovasc Diagn 1996; Supple 3: 69–72.

63. Coletti RH, Haik BJ, Wiedermann JG et al. Marked reduction in slow reflow after rotational atherectomy through use of a novel flush solution (abstract). J Invas Cardiol 1996;32.

64. Reisman M, Harms V. Guidewire bias: Potential source of complications with rotational atherectomy. Cathet Cardiovasc Diagn 1996; Supple 3:64–8.

65. Reisman M, English M, Sytman A, et al. Active guidewire technique: Using guidewire bias to assist in rotational atherectomy. J Invas Cardiol 1997; 9:30–2.

66. Mintz GS, Pichard AD, Kent KM, et al. Transcatheter device synergy: Preliminary experience with adjunct

directional coronary atherectomy following high-speed rotational atherectomy or excimer laser angioplasty in the treatment of coronary artery disease. Cathet Cardiovasc Diagn 1993; Suppl (1):37–44.

67. Reisman M, Harms V, Whitlow P, et al. Comparison of early and recent results with rotational atherectomy. J Am Coll Cardiol 1997; 29:353–7.

68. Lotan C, Rozenman Y, Weiss AT, et al. Urgent rotational ablation of a partially protected, totally occluded left main coronary artery. Cathet Cardiovasc Diagn 1996; Supple 3:78–81.

69. Cardenas JR, Strumpf RK, Heuser RR. Rotational atherectomy in restenotic lesions at the distal saphenous vein graft anastomosis. Cathet Cardiovasc Diagn. 1995; 36(1):53–7.

70. Abhyankar AD. Vaidya KA. Bernstein L. Rotational atherectomy of calcified ostial saphenous vein graft lesion with long term follow-up: A case report. Internat J Cardiol. 1995; 52(1):11–2.

71. Bowling LS, Guarneri E, Schatz RA, et al. High-speed rotational atherectomy of tortuous coronary arteries with guidewire-associated pseudostenosis. Cathet Cardiovasc Diag 1996; Supple 3:82–84.

72. Levin TN, Carroll J, and Feldman T. High speed rotational atherectomy of chronic total coronary occlusions. Cathet Cardiovasc Diag 1996; Supple 3:34–39.

73. Danchin N, Cassagnes J, Juilliere Y, et al. Balloon angioplasty versus rotational angioplasty in chronic coronary occlusions (the BAROCCO study). Am J Cardiol. 1995; 75(5):330–4.

74. Schechtmann N., Rosenblum J., Stertzer S., et al. Rotational ablation of chronic coronary occlusions. Cathet Cardiovasc Diagn 1991; 24:295–9.

75. Goldberg S, Hall P, Almagor Y, et al. Intravascular ultrasound guided rotational atherectomy of fibro-calcific plaque prior to intracoronary deployment of Palmaz-Schatz stents (abstract). J Am Coll Cardiol 1994; 23:290A.

76. Sharma SK, Duvvuri S, Kakarala V et al. Rotational atherectomy (RA) for in-stent restenosis (ISR): Intravascular ultrasound (IVUS) and quantitative coronary analysis (QCA). (abstract) Circulation 1996; 94:I–454.

77. Stone GW. Rotational atherectomy for treatment of in-stent restenosis: Role of intracoronary ultrasound guidance. Cathet Cardiovasc Diagn 1996; Supple 3:73–77.

78. David L. Fischman DL, Leon MB, et al., A Randomized Comparison of Coronary Stent Placement and Balloon Angioplasty in the Treatment of Coronary Artery Disease, N Engl J. Med, 1994; 331:496–501.

79. Patrick W. Serruys PW, de Jaegere P, Kiemeneij F, A Comparison of Balloon-Expandable-Stent Implantation with Balloon in Patients with Coronary Artery Disease, N Engl J. Med, 1994;331:489–495.

80. Abbo KM, Dooris M, Glazier S, et al. Features and outcome of no reflow after percutaneous coronary intervention. Am J Cardiol. 1995; 75(12):778–82.

81. Cohen BM, Weber VJ, Reisman M, et al. Coronary perforation complicating rotational ablation The US multicenter experience. Cathet Cardiovasc Diag 1996; Supple 3:55–59.

82. Walton AS, Pomerantsev EV, Oesterle SN, et al. Outcome of narrowing related side branches after high-speed rotational atherectomy. Am J Cardiol. 1996; 77(5):370–3.

83. Deelstra, M. H. Coronary rotational ablation: an overview with related nursing interventions. American Journal of Critical Care 1993; 2(1): 16–25; quiz 26–7.

84. Murphy MC, Hansell HN, et al. Differences in symptoms during and post-PTCA versus rotational ablation. Progress in Cardiovascular Nursing 1994; 9(2):4–9.

85. Hoffmann R, Mintz GS, Kent KM, et al. Is there an optimal therapy for calcified lesions in large vessels? Comparative acute and follow-up results of rotational atherectomy, stents or combination. J Amer Coll Cardiol 1997; 27:68A.

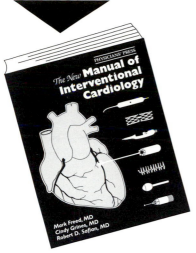
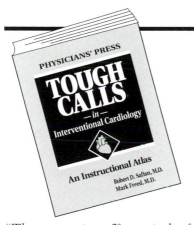
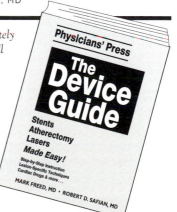

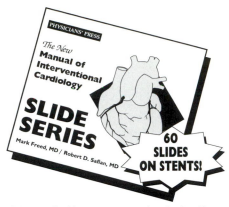
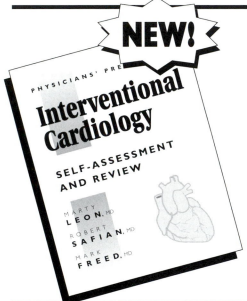
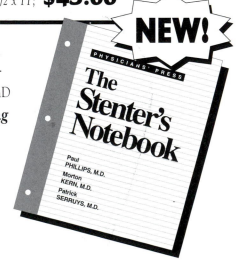

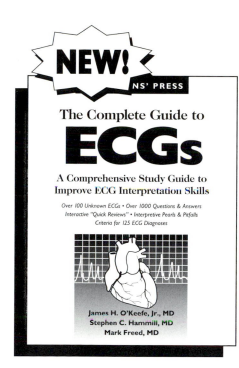

ORDERING INFORMATION
30 DAY MONEY-BACK GUARANTEE

ELECTROCARDIOGRAPHY

ITEM	DESCRIPTION	PUBLISH DATE	PRICE (US Dollars)
1	The Complete Guide to ECGs	Aug. '97	$ 49.95
2	The Complete Guide to ECGs Slide Set (100 slides)	Aug. '97	69.95
3	The ECG Criteria and ACLS Handbook	Sept. '97	12.95

INTERVENTIONAL CARDIOLOGY

ITEM	DESCRIPTION	PUBLISH DATE	PRICE (US Dollars)
4a	The New Manual of Interventional Cardiology	Update:	99.95 (hardcover)
4b	The New Manual of Interventional Cardiology	Sept. '97	84.95 (softcover)
5	The New Manual of Interventional Cardiology Slide Series (650 slides)	Nov. '96	750.00
6	Tough Calls in Interventional Cardiology	Nov. '96	129.95
7	The Device Guide	Nov. '96	39.95
8	Guide to Rotational Atherectomy	Sept. '97	59.95
9	Interventional Cardiology: Self-Assessment and Review	Sept. '97	45.00
10	The Stenter's Notebook	Sept. '97	49.95

OTHER PUBLICATIONS

ITEM	DESCRIPTION	PUBLISH DATE	PRICE (US Dollars)
11a	Essentials of Cardiovascular Medicine (unabridged)	Nov. '94	29.95
11b	Essentials of Cardiovascular Medicine (abridged)		12.95
11c	Essentials of Cardiovascular Medicine (bookset)		39.95
12	After Residency: The Young Physician's Guide to the Universe	July '97	19.95

DISCOUNT PACKAGES

ITEM	DESCRIPTION		PRICE
13	Interventional Package I: Items 4, 6, & 7		229.95* SAVE $25
14	Interventional Package II: Items 4, 5, 6, & 7		899.95* SAVE $105
15	Interventional Package III: All 6 Interventional Publications & Slides		1009.75* SAVE $150

5 Ways to Order:

Contact your local medical bookstore or:

By Phone:

(USA)
(800) 642-5494
(Outside USA)
(248) 645-6443

By Fax:

Fax order page to:
(248) 642-4949

By Internet:

www.physicianspress.com

By Mail: Mail to:

Physicians' Press
555 S. Old Woodward
Suite 1409
Birmingham, Michigan
USA 48009-6679

* Add $15 for Hard Cover Manual

§ Prices subject to change.

Sales Tax: Michigan residents add 6%; Canadian residents add 7% GST

Shipping & Handling Policy: Books & Slides are shipped immediately upon publication. It is possible to receive 2 or more shipments. **Overnight delivery available – call for charge.**

FAX / MAIL ORDER FORM

ITEM	QUANTITY	TOTAL COST
		(US Dollars)
_____	_____	_____
_____	_____	_____
_____	_____	_____

Sales Tax _____
(Michigan residents add 6%;
Canadian residents add 7% GST)

Shipping _____
(Compute shipping charge based on chart below)

TOTAL (U.S. DOLLARS) $ _____

5 Ways to Order:

Contact your local medical bookstore or:

By Phone:

(USA) (800) 642-5494
(Outside USA)
(248) 645-6443

By Fax:

Fax order page to:
(248) 642-4949

By Internet:

www.physicianspress.com

By Mail: Mail to:

Physicians' Press
555 S. Old Woodward
Suite 1409
Birmingham, Michigan
USA 48009-6679

TOTAL PURCHASE	USA UPS Ground; arrives 3–7 days	OUTSIDE USA*		
		US Postal Surface Arrives 6–8 weeks	**US Postal Air** Arrives 10-14 Days	**Express Air** UPS, FEDEX, DHL Arrives 2-5 Days
$1–35	Add $4	Add $10	Add $20	Add $30
$36–90	Add $7	Add $15	Add $30	Add $60
$91–150	Add $12	Add $20	Add $40	Add $75
$151–400	Add $14	Add $25	Add $50	Add $90
$401–750	Add $16	Add $30	Add $60	Add $120
$751+	Add $20	Add $35	Add $70	Add $150

If shipping charges exceed those listed in the chart, you will be contacted for approval prior to shipment.

For shipping outside USA, check one:
- ☐ Express Air
- ☐ US Postal Air
- ☐ US Postal Surface

☐ Check Enclosed
(US Dollars from US Bank)

☐ Bill Me

☐ Credit Card: ☐ Visa ☐ MasterCard ☐ AMEX

☐ 3-Payment Plan: Orders over $300, bill my credit card each month for 3 consecutive months.

Card No.: _____

Exp. Date: _____

Signature: _____

Name: _____
(PLEASE PRINT)

Address: _____

_____

_____

Telephone (*important*): _____

FAX (*important*): _____

e-mail _____

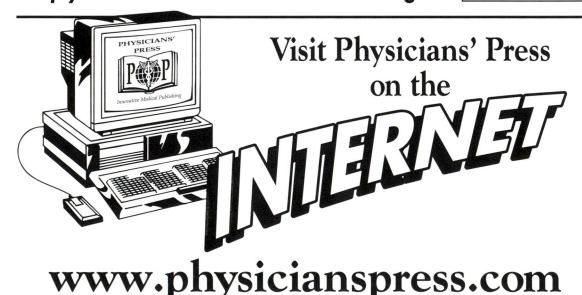